I0429721

THE TAO OF PALEO

FINDING YOUR PATH TO HEALTH AND HARMONY

BY JOE SALAMA AND JASON GOLDBERG

ORIGINAL CONCEPT BY JASON GOLDBERG

The information provided herein is only intended as anecdotal rather than advisory, and cannot substitute for the advice of a professional. Nothing herein is to be construed as an attempt to offer or render a professional medical or nutritional opinion, which cannot be done effectively without individualized consultation. Please consult with a physician before beginning any dietary or exercise regimen. Reliance on any information provided is solely at your own risk.

Published by Paleo Publishing - www.paleopublishing.com

ISBN: 1499385994
ISBN-13: 978-1499385991

Jason's Dedication: To my late grandfather Jack Goldberg, athlete, autodidact, badass, beautiful soul from a lost era. You taught me most of what I know about being a mensch. I remember you always, with love, respect, and admiration.

Joe's Dedication: To Amira and Mark, my perfect children, my students, and my teachers. You have been and will always be Yoda-level in your father's eyes. To my parents Samir and Zeinab, the best parents you could imagine. And to my Khaleesi Kathryn Lynn Haldiman, for simply being who she is.

CONTENTS

Foreword   by Jimmy Moore   Page iii

Foreword   by Darryl Edwards   Page vii

Chapter 1   Who Are You Guys and Why Did you Write This Book?   Page 1

Chapter 2   Our Story   Page 6

Chapter 3   Why?   Page 15

Chapter 4   Eat   Page 19

Chapter 5   Move   Page 47

Chapter 6   Play   Page 67

Chapter 7   Sleep   Page 80

Chapter 8   Supplements   Page 92

Chapter 9   Carbs   Page 105

Chapter 10   Protein   Page 116

Chapter 11   Fat   Page 127

Chapter 12   Breathe   Page 146

Chapter 13   Feel   Page 156

Chapter 14   The Plan   Page 161

Chapter 15   Resources   Page 186

Appendix A   Move   Page 201

Appendix B   12-Week Meal Plan   Page 209

Appendix C   Recipes, Tips and Tricks, Salad Dressing Matrix   Page 221

FOREWORD BY JIMMY MOORE

Just start hanging around the wide diversity of people in the paleo community for even a brief period of time and you'll notice something truly amazing considering this modern-day movement is not yet fully established itself and has yet to become accepted within mainstream health circles. It is comprised of real people sharing about their life experiences embodied in all the new media means of communication such as blogs, podcasts, social media, books, and more. When I first started talking about these alternative nutritional health concepts nearly a decade ago after losing 180 pounds, you could hear the crickets chirping it was so silent out there. But now if you put your ear to the ground and listen carefully, you can hear the distant roar of a large pack of wild animals galloping towards you in an unstoppable show of strength.

It's coming and you had better be ready for it.

This eclectic group of individuals describing themselves as "paleo" is unified behind the central theme of helping others find their path to health and harmony in their lives. They do this by using the talents they have been gifted with to share with everyone they can about how some rather simple changes in diet, fitness, and lifestyle can make all the difference in their overall health and general well-being. This is the overriding message that ignites the passion and zeal of the two unique individuals behind this book - Joe Salama and Jason Goldberg. If this book is any indication of the way these two fellas who are obviously friends interact in real life, then somebody needs to give them their own reality show!

I'm not quite sure how to describe the writing style of *The Tao of Paleo* for you other than to say it is arguably the most unique paleo book you'll ever read in your life. Think Beavis and Butt-Head meets The Flintstones…fire, fire, meat, meat, fire, fire, yabba dabba doo! You'll have a gay old time indeed as you work your way through the pages of this book eavesdropping in on two buds talking about the concepts of paleo while caught in a bad bromance. If you don't already know Joe and Jason, then you'll feel like you did after making it through this book. The casual conversations you're gonna see in this book are the exact kind of verbal interactions that can and must happen if paleo is ever going to penetrate our culture and become a regular part of the health conversation.

In case it's not completely obvious rather quickly in this book, Joe and Jason are completely whacked out - but in a very good way! They let you in on an intimate and critically important conversation they are having about this subject that you can tell they are super-passionate about discussing. You could almost imagine they're like that loud group of guys having dinner at the table next to you and sharing compelling information that you can't help but want to hear. What makes it so entertaining is the infusion of their larger-than-life personalities while disseminating the nuts and bolts of what it means to be paleo. One thing you won't say about this book is that it's boring. Hardly!

Reading through this book was a bit like listening to Cheech and Chong if they ever decided to adopt paleo in earnest and start talking about it. Except there's no obvious whiff of wacky weed in the air here. What you see is what you get from these two authentically paleo dudes who are taking what they know, sharing it with as many people as possible, and having some fun along the way. If everyone in the paleo community made a commitment to doing this, then the movement would make great strides faster than a speeding bullet. So you might be wondering what you've gotten yourself into with this book, huh? Well, despite my description of the whimsical nature of *The Tao of Paleo,* don't let that mislead you into thinking it's not a serious book. Humor is a fantastic way of diffusing the apprehension that some people may have regarding the paleo lifestyle and you get heaps of it throughout these pages. But what those funny bits do is open up the door of opportunity for learning, understanding, and building wisdom that can change your life just like it changed the lives of Joe Salama and Jason Goldberg.

The time for releasing your inner paleo has come. Breathe it in deeply and let it out slowly. You'll be glad you did.

Jimmy Moore
Spartanburg, South Carolina
May 2014

FOREWORD BY DARRYL EDWARDS

I am Darryl Edwards (also known as The Fitness Explorer), author of the book *Paleo Fitness* published by Ulysses Press, and founder of Fitness Explorer Training & Nutrition based in London, England. I am a certified personal trainer and paleo nutritionist who focuses on a playful approach to movement and activity, especially useful for those who don't particularly love to exercise.

I became impassioned about helping others after witnessing my own health improve significantly upon adopting an ancestral approach to well-being several years ago. With *The Tao of Paleo* it is immediately obvious that Joe Salama and Jason Goldberg, the authors behind this book, are also passionate about assisting others find a path to health. Most paleo books are focussed on food, with the premise being that if we consume foods that humans were designed to eat we will achieve optimal health and vitality. It is evident some foods nurture health while other foods will promote illness. However, this premise can sometimes fall short - but not because food isn't that significant. After all a diet based on paleo principles can deliver remarkable success when it comes to delivering weight-loss, improving health and preventing disease based on the evidence of many (myself included). There is no doubt, food is the foundation of good health.

However, man does not live on diet alone: What can we do during the rest of the day when we are not eating food that can further our pursuit of good health? What should our approach to fitness be? How should we more effectively manage stress? What else should I consider? Well *The Tao of Paleo* presents a more holistic approach to the paleo lifestyle. Not just eating, but the doing, the being, and the thinking as to what constitutes good health - for example what activities you should undertake, practical suggestions to improve the quality of your sleep, and tips on planning lifestyle changes that will make the transition easier. Once you look beyond the paleo surface and dig deeper, the realisation is that paleo is a gateway to other aspects of tuning into our bodies ancestral heritage, enabling us to make better decisions that will enhance health based on what nature intended. What is particularly interesting is the lighthearted approach in this book. Presented in a conversational style, both authors are bouncing back and forth ideas, thoughts and anecdotes offering insight into various wellbeing concepts. Joe and Jason make suggestions and offer solutions to questions often asked in the paleo community. One thing is for sure: *The Tao of Paleo* will stir you into action and spur you onto investigating broader approaches when it comes to experiencing your paleo lifestyle.

Darryl Edwards
London, England
May 2014

CHAPTER 1:
WHO ARE YOU GUYS AND WHY DID YOU WRITE THIS BOOK?

"Words are like a finger pointed at the moon. If you watch the finger, you will miss the moon." ~ Buddhist Proverb

JS: It's a valid question.

JG: Absolutely. After all, you paid good money for *The Tao of Paleo*, or maybe you are leafing through this chapter trying to decide if you want to buy. You deserve to know more about what this book is all about, and also what WE are all about.

JS: The reality is, there's nothing special about either of us. I'm from the West Coast. Jason's from back East. We're both just a couple of average Joes.

JG: Actually, you're an average Joe. I'm an average Jason.

JS: -_-

JG: Sorry.

JS: We both have regular jobs, mortgages, and typical American lives. Yeah, we both went to college. Yes, we go to the gym, but you're not going to see us curing cancer, on the cover of fitness magazines, or spot us on the red carpet at Hollywood premiers with a starlet on our arm. Neither of us are training to go fight in the Octagon. At least not this year.

JG: Both of us are single dads. We're each on the back side of forty. Also it's important to note we're not serial killers.

JS: Dude…

JG: Well, at least I'm not.

JS: There's only one thing special about us, and that's the real reason we wrote this book - because the paleo lifestyle literally changed our lives. We used to struggle with injuries and low energy. Our workouts made us tired and we didn't sleep well at night. Literally, everything we thought we knew about nutrition, exercise, and wellness - things we had been told all our lives - all of it was completely wrong.

JG: In each of our cases, someone reached out to help us make the transition to a fuller, healthier life.

JS: As I recall, in your case, that someone was me.

JG: True.

JS: Shortly after adopting the paleo lifestyle, each of us felt so energetic, so healthy and well, that we wanted to share our experiences and knowledge with our family and friends. We suddenly saw that the people close to us were living much like we were before we discovered paleo - the people we cared about were overweight, unhealthy, unhappy, unwell and in many cases on medication. We wanted to help them feel like we felt.

JG: (in a deep voice:) WE LITERALLY WANTED TO CHANGE THE WORLD!

JS: (rolls eyes) Easy there, tiger.

JG: Well, we were pretty darned excited, anyway.

JS: Yep. Jason and I started leading people toward the paleo path, hoping that we could help others. Our dear friend Karen Pendergrass, author, blogger, creator of the International Paleo Movement Group, and all-around paleo ninja, calls this "paleoing it forward."

JG: And paleo it forward we did. Both of us reached out to friends and family, offering them the same help we received. We enjoyed helping others transform their lives every bit as much as we enjoyed transforming our own.

JS: Even more. And that brings us to the purpose of this book.

JG: Exactly. We're writing this book to keep paleoing it forward to the widest possible audience. And also so I can buy a yacht. And a small Caribbean island.

JS: Goddarn it Jason…

JG: A rowboat and a few bags of dirt?

JS: Moving on. We'll do our best to lay out the basics of paleo - not just the eating but the overall philosophy from our point of view - the way we eat, the way we exercise, the way we rest, and the way we play. Should you require more information, we will also point you in the direction of terrific books, websites, podcasts, blogs, and other sources from some paleo pros who can fine-tune your transformation. At the end of the day, it will all help you find the right paleo path for you. And you might find us just a little bit entertaining along the way.

JG: Me, yes. You not so much.

JS: Moving on…

JG: There are some basic tenets of paleo that we all agree on, but in the end everyone is different. You can look at this book like the "finger pointing at the moon." We ask that you don't get absorbed in the minutiae because then you'll miss the big picture. We're pretty confident that if you look where the finger is pointing, you'll discover the paleo lifestyle that works for you. In other words, you'll see the moon, and end up in a healthier and happier place. We are going to ask something of you first, though. We need you to open your mind and realize that much of what you read here will probably be very different than what you've always believed is true. You must unlearn what you have learned.

JS: People ask us all the time if living the paleo lifestyle will make you healthier. We can only say that we - and hundreds of others we know - have lost large amounts of fat, built lean muscle, increased flexibility and functional strength, lowered blood pressure and cholesterol, increased restful sleep, and lowered stress - all of which are strongly correlated by the best science to overall health, wellness, and quality of life. And many of us have abated all symptoms of diseases that they thought they had to manage for the rest of their lives.

JG: We don't mean to suggest that this path is going to lead to rapid results for absolutely everyone.

JS: No. Everyone is different. Although we can't promise you quick results, we can promise you a path to lasting health.

JG: We are going to present you with solid science and hard evidence. However, don't be surprised when we mention some things that are contrary to what you've always heard about living in a healthy way.

JS: It's very likely that just like us, most of what you thought you knew about being healthy is wrong. We're going to fix that. Trust us, you're going to feel terrific. Your body will get leaner. You will feel more energetic. You will sleep more soundly. You will manage stress better. Each day will begin to look more like an adventure and less like a chore. We wrote *The Tao of Paleo* to paleo it forward to you - to help you live a healthier, happier, and more satisfying life.

JG: In short, to help you become what we like to call "PAF." That means Paleo as Fu...

JS: Yo! Jason! This is a G-rated book!

JG: Oh yeah. Sorry. :(

CHAPTER TWO: OUR STORY

"Tell me what you eat, and I'll tell you what you are." ~ *Anthelme Brillat-Savarin*

JS: Yep. He's right, that's for sure.

JG: Who's right?

JS: Anthelme Brillat-Savarin.

JG: Anthem Brillo who??

JS: (Sigh) Look up, Jason.

JG: I can't look up. We're two-dimensional.

JS: Look at the top of the page, dude. At the quote. See it now? The guy was a famous French chef from the eighteenth century, and he basically said you are what you put into your body.

JG: You're right. He is right.

JS: Unfortunately, using Brillat-Savarin's axiom, people who eat the Standard American Diet are unhealthy, because they eat things that are innately unhealthy for humans to eat.

JG: Agreed, Joe, and until recently, we were both just like them. We ate the Standard American Diet and we got the standard American results - poor health.

JS: We also followed the "standard," of what we had always been told was healthy exercise - lots of cardio to burn calories and to build a healthy heart. If Brillat-Savarin were a trainer, he probably would have said something like "tell me how you exercise, and I'll tell you why you feel like garbage." I was a big runner - covering miles and miles each week.

JG: I used to run thirty miles a week. If I didn't, I just knew I would morph into the pudgy, middle-aged guy I dreaded becoming. Not to mention I would drop dead of a massive heart attack.

JS: I rarely lifted heavy weights. I didn't want to get too bulky. Weight lifters were big beefy guys in tank tops and stretchy shorts who waddled around injecting each other with syringes.

JG: I never walked. Walking was a waste of time. It was for old people, or people who couldn't run.

JS: Back on the dietary front, I ate "healthy" food - lots of whole grains, "heart-healthful" oils and polyunsaturated fats, and lean protein. I ate pasta and rice, and I drank 6-8 glasses of water every day.

JG: I was partial to eating those protein bars chock-full of whey or soy protein, and a whole bunch of ingredients with six syllables and lots of x's and y's in the name. Polysorbalox Dylathanol was one of my favorites.

JS: Dude, you just made that up.

JG: True, but doesn't it sound delicious?

JS: No. I was putting away those bars like nobody's business too. Anyway, even though I was "eating healthy" and "exercising right," I felt terrible. I had been diagnosed with ADHD and it was getting worse. I couldn't stay on task or concentrate on anything for very long without my medication - prescription amphetamines.

JG: I slept terribly, no more than six hours per night. I tossed and turned and woke up constantly. I would get out of bed in the morning exhausted and sore. I used to dread going to sleep.

JS: I had awful seasonal allergies that just seemed to get worse every year. I was developing digestion issues. Physically, my muscle tone was poor and I had a layer of fat around my waist that wouldn't go away no matter how much I ran. I was addicted to running and I felt great as long as my body was pumping adrenaline and endorphins into my system, but as soon as I stopped I felt terrible…and I didn't even know it because it was a gradual onset and progression of malaise.

JG: I had the same ring of chub around my belly. I thought I could get rid of it by working out harder. I'd go to the gym and do an hour of circuit training, never stopping for a rest or a drink. I'd lie on my dining room floor afterward, nauseous, thinking to myself that this was the price I needed to pay to stay in shape. Later, I'd have a salad with a small scoop of tuna or a protein bar, convinced that if I just restricted calories and trained harder, I'd have the fit body I really wanted.

JS: I was running half and full marathons, and I absolutely LIVED on "healthy" grains. Meanwhile, my ADHD wasn't getting any better. My ability to plan and execute projects was only functional because of my meds, which I loathed taking because of the unpleasant side effects. The hearing in my right ear was deteriorating and I just chalked it up to getting older. After all, things just start going downhill after 35, right? That's just life.

JG: High blood pressure and heart disease ran in my family, and I had always been pre-hypertensive, no matter how "fit" I was or how "healthy" my diet was. And it seemed to be getting worse - my systolic pressure would creep up into the low 140s if I had a rough few days and I figured it was just a matter of time before I needed to look at medication - which by the way, would have put me out of my job, because we aren't allowed to take it. My "healthy" diet was hard on my digestion. I had frequent and embarrassing bouts of gas and indigestion. After a protein bar I typically steered clear of human company for at least an hour or so.

JS: I just got to a point where I was no longer satisfied with the concept of my life deteriorating. I was ready to find a different path - a better Tao.

JG: Let's talk about what that means. It's the first time we've mentioned it, and it must be important because it's in the title of this book.

JS: "Tao" (pronounced "Dow") in Chinese philosophy implies a way, or a path...but it's much more than that.

JG: It means a code, a way of being, that puts you in harmony with yourself, your surroundings, and the universe.

JS: Of course, there are different "Taos" for different things, and for different people.

JG: Agreed. Just like paleo, which is isn't a cookbook, a diet, an exercise plan, or a fad, and it isn't the same for any two people.

JS: Nope, paleo is a path, a way, a method to bring your body and yourself into harmony with your surroundings and the universe.

JG: In other words, it's a Tao - *The Tao of Paleo*. Now let's get back to talking about how you found your Tao.

JS: A good friend of mine, a fellow named David Storey, had suggested to me that I try paleo.

JG: As I recall the story, Joe, he suggested you try it eight or nine times before you finally listened to him.

JS: Jason…

JG: Stubborn dude that Joe Salama. Probably was even worse when he had ADHD.

JS: May I finish?

JG: By all means.

JS: Anyway, I decided to give it a try. I jumped into it head first not knowing that much about it until after I started. Although I had a bit of a rough start with carb and glucose withdrawal, it wasn't long before I was feeling very different. I had lots of energy. I was sleeping soundly. By then I had made my way through *Good Calories, Bad Calories* by Gary Taubes, and was completely disgusted with grains. I couldn't believe what I had been doing to my body by eating them. My allergies also started to abate – both my food and seasonal allergies. One day, I finished a project at work in record time, and absolutely nailed it. I thought to myself "thank goodness for my ADHD medicine" then I realized I hadn't taken it. Major epiphany.

JG: Go Joe!!

JS: (bowing) Thank you. I started to change the way I exercised, too. No more steady state cardio - I learned that it just increased my body's production of cortisol, a hormone that caused me to retain belly fat and actually burn muscle. In retrospect, this explained what I wasn't getting thinner despite logging so many miles each week. Instead, I started a paleo regimen of weightlifting, leisurely walking, and interval training.

JG: You started exercising and eating like humans are meant to do. You got yourself in harmony with yourself and your universe. You found your Tao.

JS: Exactly. The results were stunning and they happened quickly. Within four months, my body became leaner and I rapidly built aesthetically pleasing muscle. My aches and pains vanished. And people noticed. My friends started to tell me I looked fifteen years younger. I was so excited about paleo I wanted to start paleoing it forward to share what I'd experienced. I started to do what David did - I began to tell people about my transformation, and I recommended that they give it a try. Now, two and a half years later, I have over 600 converts under my belt.

JG: It must be pretty crowded under there.

JS: There's a lot more room available after all the fat loss. Let's talk about you.

JG: This is where I come into the story. Joe mentioned to me on several occasions that I should try the paleo lifestyle, and I politely ignored him. After all, I was fit. I was healthy. I was a former college athlete. I knew what I was doing.

JS: How did that work for you?

JG: Not too well. But it took a major event to get me to finally listen to Joe and give paleo a try.

JS: It was a girl.

JG: Yep.

JS: It's always a girl with you.

JG: (moving fingers and thumb in a talking motion) Joe, this is what you are doing. (pressing fingers together) This is what I want you to do.

JS: Ok, ok. Fine. Go ahead.

JG: Anyway, I was totally in love with Rachel. I thought I had finally met "The One." For several months we spent every waking minute together. In my heart I just knew we were going to live happily ever after.

JS: Until she dumped you.

JG: Via email no less. At any rate, this very unpleasant experience forced me into a lot of serious self-reflection. I realized I wasn't just unhappy, but that I wasn't feeling very well either. All my "fitness" and all my "healthy eating" wasn't making me very fit or healthy. I decided to make a radical change. I needed to find a new Tao.

JS: You decided to listen to me.

JG: I decided to try a 30-day course of strict paleo. It was as if my body had been waiting for years for me to figure it out. I was rewarded with almost instant results. I developed a steady reserve of calm, clear energy. My sleep improved dramatically. My stomach settled down. After the first 30 days I decided to change my workout regimen.

JS: Just like I did.

JG: Exactly. I dropped the cardio and shortened up my circuit workouts to a more reasonable twenty minutes or so. I started lifting heavy weights and added walking and sprinting to my schedule. Combined with the dietary changes, it was like alchemy. The fat melted off my waist. Instead of feeling exhausted during and after my workouts, I felt energized by them. I developed amazing flexibility and suddenly I could do headstands, handstands, cartwheels, you name it. I caught my reflection in the mirror one morning and I actually saw my abs. I almost cried.

JS: You cried over your own abs. That might be the funniest thing I've ever heard. And also the saddest.

JG: Laugh if you will, Joe. It takes a real man to cry. Over his abs.

JS: Back on topic, please. Tell the blood pressure story.

JG: Sure. About six months after starting paleo, I was walking through the supermarket and I saw one of those fancy blood pressure machines in the pharmacy section. I figured, what the heck, I'd see how my BP was doing. After all, I felt pretty good, and maybe the ol' blood pressure had gone down a few points.

JS: You were in for a surprise.

JG: I sure was. My systolic pressure had gone down by thirty points, my diastolic by fifteen. I thought it was a mistake. I must have spent a half an hour at that machine, testing my blood pressure again and again. It was true. My blood pressure was normal. No medication. Just clean eating, good rest, and proper exercise. My doctor tested me half a dozen times at my next physical a few weeks later. He didn't believe it was possible.

JS: But there it was.

JG: That was the icing on the cake. Or the grass-fed butter on the steak. That's much more paleo.

JS: Anyway, that's the story of who we are - and much more importantly, what *The Tao of Paleo* did for us.

JG: We just want to remind you that our stories aren't rare in the paleo community. Not by a long shot. WE are but two of thousands who have undergone this fundamental metamorphosis of body, mind and spirit. We finally made the decision to stop fighting against millions of years of evolution and start eating, sleeping, playing, and working out like humans are meant to do. We decided to follow our Tao - to be in harmony with ourselves and our surroundings.

JS: That's right, and it's important to remember that you can make the same choice as we did. If you find your own Tao of Paleo, it's a cinch that you can achieve similarly positive results.

JG: Maybe even better.

JS: Absolutely. And now that you know who we are, and what we've done, it's time to start telling you what The Tao of Paleo is all about.

JG: Hold on – it's going to be the ride of your life!

JS: Always with the drama. This is a book, not a roller coaster.

JG: Thanks, Buzz Killian.

JS: -_-

CHAPTER THREE: WHY?

"I think, therefore I am." ~ Rene Descartes

JS: You think, therefore you are Rene Descartes?

JG: (ignoring him) We figure the first question you're going to ask us after "What is *The Tao of Paleo*?" is "Why *The Tao Paleo*?"

JS: This whole line of questioning usually starts with something like: "Hmm…paleo…is that the same thing as the caveman diet?"

JG: And your answer?

JS: Well…yes and no.

JG: You sound like a lawyer.

JS: I am a lawyer. But I am still a nice guy.

JG: I think that's an open question. It's definitely true that there are issues with the concept of paleo being "the caveman diet."

JS: The caveman diet or ancestral diet premise asserts that we should follow the paleo lifestyle because it is based on the way our ancient forefathers lived. Specifically, that we should eat the foods that our ancestors - Paleolithic man - ate. Speaking loosely, we mean from 100,000 years ago to about 10,000 years ago - before the agricultural revolution took place and before the Neolithic era started.

JG: How do we know what people ate 100,000 years ago? I haven't seen too many Paleolithic-era videos on YouTube.

JS: We logically assume that they didn't eat many grains because most cultures did not develop the tools needed to process grains until approximately 10,000 years ago.

JG: We can also analyze bone samples and determine how much protein our ancestors ate. We do know for sure that Paleolithic man didn't eat chemicals and processed foods because they didn't exist back then. It's important to realize though, at the end of the day, we can't tell you with precision exactly what our ancestors ate.

Joe, let's talk about the disease theory.

JS: The theory goes that our ancestors did not have many of the diseases we have today, like heart disease, obesity, hypertension, type 2 diabetes, epithelial cell cancers, autoimmune diseases, and osteoporosis, and that they did not have these diseases because of what they ate.

JG: Clearly, archeologists have discovered the chart room from Paleolithic Memorial Hospital. How else would we know what diseases our ancestors had?

JS: Well, there is no evidence of those diseases in the fossil record or among present day hunter-gatherer societies.

JG: Ok, but just because our ancestors didn't have certain diseases and ate a certain way doesn't mean that the reason they didn't have those diseases is because they ate that way. Scientists refer to this as "correlation" as opposed to "causation." If you sleep with your clothes on and wake up with a headache, it doesn't mean that the reason you woke up with a headache is because you didn't find your favorite Batman pajamas the night before.

JS: Are they footsie pajamas, Jason?

JG: It's not necessary to delve into the details of my pajamas. The point we're making is that we can't say for sure exactly what our ancestors ate, or the reason for the absence of certain illnesses present today at epidemic levels. And to be perfectly honest, we don't really care. We're going to leave that debate to the anthropologists, archeologists, and all the other people who wear fuzzy sweaters and jackets with elbow patches and smoke pipes.

JS: Bingo. The ancestral diet debate is one reason we have a problem with the word *paleo*. We're going to keep calling this lifestyle paleo in this book as a convention, but you might as well call it the Awesomesauce lifestyle, or the Magenta Wombat lifestyle.

JG: When we start explaining to people that the question of whether or not this is an authentic ancestral diet is something like the question "Could Batman could beat up a Tyrannosaurus?" we usually get the questions "Why eat this way? Why LIVE this way?"

JS: The answer is: Because thousands of people who have found their paleo Tao have achieved unbelievable health benefits. They no longer suffer from the diseases we mentioned. Their blood work and body chemistry is exemplary. They sleep well. They look younger. They feel incredibly energetic. They have lean, strong, attractive bodies.

JG: Why eat this way? Why LIVE this way? It's very simple: Because it works.

JS: After you read this book, hopefully you'll begin to seek out more information on the paleo lifestyle. There's no doubt you'll discover endless iterations of the debate on the authenticity of paleo.

JG: Did our Paleolithic ancestors eat this? Did they eat that? Did they run long distances or sprint short ones? Did they cultivate grains or simply forage them occasionally? It's all a very interesting debate, but on a practical level, we don't think it really matters. What matters is that it works.

JS: Maybe you find yourself asking "Wait a second - do I really want to try to find my paleo Tao if I can't be sure that the paleo lifestyle means living in authentic, strict accordance with the ways of my Paleolithic ancestors?"

JG: That depends. Do you want to feel better than you did at 25 years old, improve your overall health and energy, enjoy restful and refreshing sleep, help insulate yourself from a horde of diseases and conditions, and look younger, fitter, and more attractive?

JS: If you do - isn't it worth trying what we recommend in this book for 30 days to see if these claims are legit?

JG: We see you nodding your heads yes.

JS: See? We knew you were smart the second you bought this book.

CHAPTER FOUR: EAT

"Have a big dinner, have a light snack
If you don't like it, you can't send it back
Just eat it, eat it, eat it, eat it." ~ Weird Al

JG: It's all about food. Real food, unprocessed natural food. We should be having another guest arrive any minute now...

[knocking on the door]

JS: Didn't know we had a door in this book. How do I open it?

JG: I think you just type "opens door."

JS: [opens door] Dude, that worked!

GG: Hi Jason and Joe! I am Gary Grainiak and I LOVE GRAINS! I start out the morning with a huge vat of oat bran cereal and a bagel, I have a hearty sandwich from Subway for lunch with a bag of Sun Chips, and for dinner I have chicken with corn and whole grain rice!! And by the way, I feel AWESOME! (smiles big)

JG: Shall we shoot him now, or wait till later?

JS: Shoot him now! Shoot him now! Just kidding. We aren't here to kill off our fictitious characters, we are here to help people. Ok it's time to talk about FOOD - specifically, what should a Tao seeker eat, and what should a Tao seeker avoid?

GG: GREAT! To be honest this is the make-it-or-break-it chapter for me. I don't like the idea of restricted diet at all, but I am trying to keep an open mind here. So what's on the menu?

JG: No, wait, Joe lied. First we need to talk about *why* things are on, or off, the menu. Some of you just want to hear the bottom line. "Tell me what to do!" you're shouting to yourself as you smack yourself in the head with this book.

JS: We don't advise that, especially if you downloaded the electronic version.

JG: Others need to understand a little more about why. We're going to talk a little about the science behind the food choices and we're going to start by telling you to eat a lot of food. Paleo is not a calorie restriction diet designed to make people lose weight simply by depriving the body and making it burn stored fat.

JS: That's right. Good call, Jason. You're most certainly going to eat a lot of food, and you're not going to count calories. Instead, you'll focus on eating the RIGHT foods.

JG: Exactly.

JS: We'll divide foods into three categories: the ones that help your body function, the ones that hurt your body function, and the ones that are ok in moderation. We need to understand what makes the good foods good and the bad ones bad. The YES list is comprised of the foods that give us what we need to operate most effectively - the foods that give us all the essential nutrients we need. The NO list is a list of the all the foods the have a net negative effect on your body. They cause inflammation, auto-immune disorders, insulin insensitivity, contain toxins, and otherwise wreak havoc on normal bodily functions. The MODERATION list is comprised of foods that are fine in occasional doses, but can be problematic if you eat them too often or in too large a quantity.

GG: Ok, well, who decides what is on which list? When do we get to eat grains? (pulls out baguette and starts chomping away)

JG: We use a Ouija board.

JS: Not the Ouija board again. Please.

JG: Just kidding. Science decides. Research and countless studies back up all the statements about food that we make in this chapter.

JS: Here's the nutshell: Meat, veggies, and fruits are IN.

GG: That was easy. A bit anti-climactic if you ask me. If that's it, why do we need a whole chapter for it then? Why such a big fuss?

JG: Because 90% of what most Americans eat is OFF the menu. Because there are a few items that are on the NO list even though they are veggies. And because we still need to go through *why* for each of the items on the NO list.

GG: Ok, all so I assume that packaged food is off the menu - not brain surgery there.

JS: Not necessarily - packaged might be ok - if raw almonds are packaged it's fine, but unpackaged beans are off the menu. Packaging is not a good test for - we need an adjective here - for paleosity.

JG: Paleosity? Sounds a bit pretentious.

GG: *Wait!!! Beans are NOT ok? I thought they were a good source of protein!!*

JG: So is human feces, but that doesn't mean you should eat it. And they actually aren't a good source of protein.

JS: Wow Jason, could you have found a more disgusting example?

GG: *Ok, I'll bite. Why are beans off the menu?*

JS: Not just beans - all legumes.

GG: *What the heck is a legume?*

JS: Beans, peas, peanuts…they are the plants that are part of certain scientific families or the fruit or seeds of those plants.

GG: *So why are they off the menu? I thought peanut butter sandwiches were the healthiest thing ever. What could be better for you than grains and peanuts??*

JG: Legumes contain lectins, saponins, and other natural compounds that were evolved by plants to fight off insects. These substances increase intestinal permeability and may trigger your immune system to turn against your own body, leading to autoimmune diseases. They also contain "anti-nutrient" substances like protease inhibitors and phytic acid - which prevent the proper absorption of B vitamins, iron, zinc, copper, and calcium in the intestines.

JS: As a special bonus, they also give you gas.

GG: *Wow. Ok, so no legumes…that's not the end of the world. And I know my wife Gloria Grainiak will appreciate the gas reduction.*

JG: They are off the paleo menu, yes. If you are absolutely passionate about having legumes, try adding them back in

small amounts after totally abstaining for thirty days in order to test out how your body responds. Yes, I know a couple of paleo people that decided to eat peanut butter every couple of weeks and are otherwise 100% paleo. At least they have made an informed choice. Everyone, after all, eventually adapts the paleo template. They find their own Tao.

JS: Look at it like a control/variable experiment. You see how you do with a clean slate and then you can measure the effect of each additional food you reintroduce. We will tell you, however, that legumes are not a good choice for most humans unless they are sprouted or fermented, both of which alter some of the problematic compounds. You're likely to feel much better without legumes.

JG: Exactly. For example, some people think that beans make them feel good but have never gone without them for long enough for them to realize that beans actually make them feel horrible. This is another example of the unfortunate truth that most people have no idea how great their bodies were designed to feel.

GG: Hold on a second…Yeah yeah, sure, and of course, I only have to give you my firstborn child, Gustav Grainiak, in order to buy the special paleo foods you want to sell me in order to feel so awesome. I'm on to your game, pyramid marketing boy. I used to sell Amway, after all.

JG: You can keep Gustav. We don't want to sell you anything. There is no secret fat-burning elixir or magic salve or any snake oil to buy. Maybe you should consider the idea that if someone - or in this case thousands of someones - are so excited about something, and they don't want your money or anything else from you, it might be a good sign that there may be some truth to what they are saying. Let's get back to the NO list. Joe, you handle this one. Did you get the anvil we ordered from Acme Anvil Company?

JS: Right here. Meep Meep.

JG: (makes whistling noise like falling anvil) HERE IT COMES! AAAAAAAA!!!!

JS: GRAINS!

(a moment of silence passes)

GG: Grains! Finally! I thought you forgot about them! "Ohhhhh Beautiful, for spacious skies, for amber waves of grain…"

JS: We probably should have started the NO list with grains. Maybe I will go back and edit this chapter later. If there were a big bad wolf…

JG: I would barbecue him, and eat his liver with some fava beans and a nice Chianti. Oops. Strike that. No beans, no Chianti. But I would eat him for sure. Wolf meat is totally paleo.

JS: Well, yes, sure, but I meant to stay that if there ever were a paleo public enemy number one, it would be grains. Grains are bad news. Yes, this includes corn. Drop them like a bad habit.

JG: (starts singing) Fight the power! We've got to fight the powers that be!

JS: Please stop.

JG: OK. But I know what time it is. You realize Gary that we are talking about granola, cereal, doughnuts, bagels, crackers and bread, right? They are big NOs. No as in non, nein, nay, and no way, José.

GG: They are OUT?!?!?

JS: Out like polyester and pleated pants.

GG: *Why are grains paleo public enemy number one?*

JS: Here's the ancestral diet theory answer. In the last 10,000 years, roughly the time we've cultivated grains, humans haven't fully evolved the necessary biology to digest them. But as you know, we have more than a couple of issues with the ancestral diet theory, starting with the fact that we don't care about it. So screw the theory, let's talk about the science. Let's start with gluten.

GG: *I knew you two were up to something. You ain't gluten nobody.*

JG: Gary, not everyone reading this has seen Trading Places.

GG: *My point here is that I have no idea what the hell gluten is - although I have seen that word a lot lately.*

JS: Gluten is the protein in wheat. You have seen that word a lot because it's been in the news so much lately. 10-15% of Americans have either celiac disease or are seriously gluten-intolerant.

GG: *Ok, but that's not me. I like my bagels. In fact, I love them. In fact, when I am feeling a little, ummmm, lonely, like when my wife is away...*

JG: Oh gosh, I am gonna be sick. Please, please stop, right now.

GG: *Sorry. I really, really like bagels, though.*

JS: So did I. But there is still a large likelihood - probably over 90% - that you and gluten don't get along.

GG: *What does that mean?*

JS: Well, gluten - after you eat it - breaks down, in part, into this other protein called alpha-gliadin.

GG: *Sounds like a character from Lord of the Rings.*

JS: And when the alpha-gliadin is in your system, your body sees it as an undigestible foreign threat. It opens up the intestinal walls to allow your immune system to enter your intestine to help fight off this invader.

The result is a condition called leaky gut. And it can contribute to a whole mess of auto-immune diseases - Hashimoto's, ADHD, rheumatoid arthritis, multiple sclerosis…the list goes on. Up to 200 different diseases have been linked to leaky gut.

GG: *That doesn't sound like fun. So are gluten-free products paleo?*

JG: Depends on the product. If it's a gluten free steak, it's good. There shouldn't be any wheat in the meat to begin with. However, if it has a list of ingredients five inches long containing chemicals you have never heard of, it's not paleo. Chemicals, additives, preservatives, food colorings - all that stuff is not paleo. The list of common additives to processed foods - soy lecithin, yellow #5, potassium benzoate, guar gum, and others - is almost endless. Stay away from anything and everything that you don't recognize. Most of the commercially available gluten free products are mostly composed of these artificial ingredients that would be right at home in a chemistry set. Your body is not a lab experiment, so you can't pump it full of chemicals and expect it to function correctly. End of rant.

GG: *Ok, so gluten is the reason not to eat grains?*

JS: One of the big ones, yes. Modern grains have been engineered to grow in soil that is devoid of most nutrients and contain much more gluten than ever. Grains also make up a larger portion of the standard American diet each year. These are two of the reasons why there has been such a dramatic increase in all autoimmune diseases and incidents of celiac disease.

Why is this true? There's a lot of blame to go around. You can blame the food pyramid, which is a great guide to achieving obesity and ill health. You can blame the food industry which continues to churn out more processed, grain-based psuedo-food every year. You can blame the medical community, which seems to have a bizarre fascination with grains and fiber. You can blame the government farm subsidies, which make unhealthy food cheaper and more available than healthy food. Before you blame everything else, though, you need to look in the mirror. The biggest share of blame belongs to we consumers for not bothering to learn what their food is doing to us. It's costing people their health - and in many cases their lives.

JG: Hey this book is supposed to be funny. That was more heavy stuff. The least you could have done was start singing *Man In The Mirror* **and grab your crotch.**

JS: OK, well, end of MY rant. Joke time. Did you hear the one about the rabbi, the priest, and the deaf guy?

JG: No.

JS: Neither did the deaf guy.

JG: Don't quit your day job. You're annoying enough as it is. I'd toss rotten tomatoes at you, but they're nightshades and they might cause inflammation.

JS: Thanks.

GG: Ok, but what about corn? It doesn't have any wheat - or gluten - if I understand you correctly.

JG: That's right.

GG: Why is it on the no list? Isn't it a vegetable?

JS: No. It's a grain. Insect food.

GG: That's harsh. I love popcorn, and corn on the cob.

JS: Unless you're a bug, it doesn't like you.

GG: What am I, a rhinoceros beetle? You're going to have to explain.

JS: Ok, fine. So grain-based carbohydrates, like those in corn, or a bagel, or a baguette, turn into sugar when they come into contact with your saliva.

GG: Sugar?

JG: You got it. So when you eat a handful of popcorn, you are essentially eating a mouthful of sugar, because your body digests it and turns it into sugar super-duper quick.

GG: Yuck.

JG: Not at all! It tastes delicious and therefore must be good for you! Plus we have to think of the poor dental industry that needs us to eat lots of grains…

GG: Point made. So I assume that grains - including corn and rice - can be just as addictive as sugar, even if they don't contain gluten?

JS: Yep. Not only that, but because our body converts these grain-based carbohydrates into sugar so quickly and easily, they also result in increased…

JG: DUM DUM DUM…

JS: …stored body fat.

GG: Doesn't your body need carbohydrates for energy, like, I've heard of this thing called…umm…glycogen?

JG: We do need carbs, and you're right. Our body stores glucose obtained from eating carbs in the liver and the muscles in the form of glycogen, a starchy substance used to fuel intense physical effort. We'll discuss this in more detail in our chapter called *Carbs*.

What we will mention here is that eating too many grain-based or sugary carbs causes a massive overload of sugar-glucose, to be more precise - in your body. To stop you from keeling over dead from elevated blood glucose, your body releases a hormone called insulin. The insulin shuttles some of the glucose into the liver and muscles to be stored as the glycogen you mentioned, and some of it is absorbed into the cells. However, it doesn't take much of this type of rocket fuel to fill the glycogen tanks. Even worse, when you eat a diet composed mostly of grains and sugary carbs, the receptors in your body's cells are so used to being flooded with insulin, they don't absorb, or "uptake," the glucose very well.

As a result, when you habitually ingest meals biased toward grains and sugary carbs, there's a huge amount of glucose left over in your bloodstream. Too much glucose is toxic to your body, so something has to be done with the extra.

JS: What happens to all that extra glucose is, it gets stored as…

JG: DUM DUM DUM…

JS: …fat.

GG: So…too much sugar makes you fat? And grains, they turn into too much sugar once you eat them, and they make you fat too?!?

JG: And if they weigh more than a duck, they are made of wood, and you are a witch.

JS: Shut it Jason. Bravo, Grainiak! Bravissimo!! (claps)

JG: Dude, why are you clapping? This is a book. No one can hear you.

GG: *Anything else about grains?*

JS: Yep. They cause systemic inflammation.

GG: *My organs get inflamed?*

JG: People think that they are losing weight the first couple of days after beginning to eat in accordance with the paleo template - but it's often just the reduction in the inflammation in their body.

GG: *I can think of an organ that could use a little inflammation.*

JS: Once you fix your diet, your body will function the way it was designed to. Your testosterone levels will naturally rise and your organ will work better. Bonus.

GG: *Wow, that's a major selling point right there. My organ is totally out of tune. Anything else bad about grains?*

JG: Yes. They all contain lectins and phytic acid in far greater amounts than legumes. As we mentioned, those are anti-nutrients.

GG: *That sounds like a bogus word, like anti-happiness or something. What the hell is an anti-nutrient?*

JS: They prevent the proper absorption of vitamins and minerals in your body. So the amount of vitamins and minerals you need from food to function perfectly actually decreases just by dropping grains from your plate.

GG: Ok, but don't we get vitamins and minerals from cereals and grains?

JG: No. Remember, the anti-nutrients prevent our bodies from absorbing whatever healthy stuff is in cereal and grains, and they don't contain anything essential for humans anyhow. Even brown rice, whole grain rice, and corn - none of which have gluten - contain loads of phytic acid. Ironically, even when grains are fortified with vitamins and minerals, the phytic acid in the grains prevents the body from absorbing most of them. Although grains are a source of the macronutrient carbohydrate, you can get your carbs without eating grains by eating fruit and starchy vegetables. Again, we'll hit that subject in-depth in the chapter *Carbs*.

GG: What about fiber? Don't we need fiber? Doesn't a lack of fiber cause stuff like diverticulitis? Don't we need fiber to poop regularly, lower cholesterol, and reduce our chances of getting diseases?

JS: No one knows what causes diverticulitis, except that stress and poor colon health contribute to it. If you have a healthy gut, you will poop as much as you need to. Excessively high cholesterol is another issue, and we will talk about that in the chapter *Fats*. Suffice to say that grains are not a good answer.

JG: As for fiber, there's plenty of it in green vegetables and fruits. One apple, one pear, or a cup of blueberries has just as much, if not more, fiber than two slices of whole wheat bread. Avocados are also an excellent source. So no, you don't need grains for fiber.

GG: Is that all you guys have to say about grains?

JS: No. Here's another fun fact for you: Many grains, like quinoa for example, also contain saponins.

GG: *I have no idea what those are.*

JG: **Saponins are chemicals evolved to protect plants from microbes and insects by dissolving the cell membranes of the potential threat.**

JS: Like a phaser in Star Trek.

JG: **Saponins are also in legumes, by the way, and they are another reason we have both grains and legumes on the paleo NO list.**

JS: They contain protease inhibitors which resist digestion and can create an imbalance in the digestive enzymes. This can result in leaky gut - we already discussed what a bad deal that is.

GG: *Wow.*

JG: **I'd like to mention a recent scientific study, led by Dr. Rajiv Chowdhury of Cambridge University. The details were published in the *Annals of Internal Medicine*. We'll be talking about this huge mega-study a lot in this book, but one of the major findings suggests that the primary culprit in heart disease and stroke is a diet high in sugary carbs and grains.**

GG: *Ok Thomas Dolby, you're blinding me with science. My head is starting to throb.*

JS: Yep. Let's review what we've laid out so far. No grains, no beans, no chemicals, food coloring, and unrecognized additives…

JG: **Dude, what's wrong with Gary?**

JS: I don't know. It looks like we overloaded his brain. He's starting to zombie out.

JG: No way! A grain zombie?!? They eat grains AND brains!!

GG: *(starts moaning, reaches for Jason's head, chanting) Grains! Brains!*

JS: Oh snap. I left my shotgun in the trunk.

JG: Hold on! I have a package of saltine crackers they threw in with lettuce-wrapped grass-fed burger at the deli!! It's in my backpack. If. I. Can. Just. Reach. It. In. Time. AHA! Got 'em!! Here! Grainiak! Suck on these!

GG: *(Gobbblegoobblegobble) Wow. My head is still killing me! What happened?*

JG: You almost morphed into a zombie, and forced me to shoot you in the head.

GG: *Oh.*

JS: Man, that was a close call. Ok, where were we? What's next on the NO list?

JG: "Natural" flavors. (snicker, sarcastic sneer)

JS: Thanks Jason. Natural flavors are basically anything extracted from nature that have not been shown to harm people. Here's the official definition of a natural flavor: "The essential oil, oleoresin, essence or extractive, protein hydrolysate, distillate, or any product of roasting, heating or enzymolysis, which contains the flavoring constituents derived from a spice, fruit or fruit juice, vegetable or vegetable juice, edible yeast, herb, bark, bud, root, leaf or similar plant material, meat, seafood, poultry, eggs, dairy products, or fermentation products thereof, whose significant function in food is flavoring rather than nutritional."

JG: Sounds "natural" to me.

GG: *That's good right? It's not artificial? Like vanilla extract?*

JG: **No. It's still created in a lab. You should be concerned that they don't tell you exactly what it is on the label. If something contains vanilla extract, then it should say "vanilla extract" on the label and not "natural flavors." You want to know what is making your food with natural flavors smell like vanilla? Look up "castoreum" on the internet. You'll never touch the stuff ever again. Stay away from natural flavors as you would "artificial flavors." It's the same game of chemical roulette.**

GG: *Ok, no natural OR artificial flavors. What's next?*

JS: Processed foods. They come in all shapes and sizes, and lots of them have grains or some element of grains as their main ingredients. Typical examples are things like potato chips, noodles, crackers, and frozen dinners. There are other processed foods that are nominally meat based, but they are just as bad. For example, Spam and hot dogs. Learn to look at ingredient lists before you buy. Don't take anything for granted. A product with more than a handful of ingredients, or ingredients you don't recognize, is a big, fat, NO. Remember the study we mentioned earlier. A diet high in the bad carbs present in these foods raises the risk of heart disease.

JG: **I quote the estimable Dr. Chowdhury, who said in a recent interview: "It's the high carbohydrate or sugary diet that should be the focus of dietary guidelines."**

JS: That's a perfect segue to our next NO - processed sugars.

GG: *Ok, that's an obvious one - so of course, natural brown sugar is ok, but white sugar is bad.*

JG: **Have you ever seen a brown sugar tree?**

GG: *Ok fine, so brown sugar is processed too. Are there any sweeteners that are not processed?*

JG: Sure. Maple syrup, honey, and molasses. Most of what you see in packaged food, though, isn't natural. High fructose corn syrup is probably the most common sweetener present in food today. The only thing worse than actual corn is the processed sugary syrup derived from corn.

GG: What about agave nectar? Isn't it supposed to be healthy?

JS: So are grains. The truth is that agave nectar is worse than high fructose corn syrup - it's a super-concentrated form of fructose. Very not good.

GG: Damn.

JG: The truth is, it's best to avoid processed sweeteners altogether and to limit your intake of natural sweeteners to very small amounts. All of these sweeteners will cause large blood sugar spikes, resulting in the insulin reaction we discussed earlier. Of course, the end result is...

JS: DUM DUM DUM...

JG: ...more body fat. And an increased likelihood of heart disease.

GG: How about artificial sweeteners, like aspartame, or Splenda?

JS: Oh yeah. Those are good for you.

GG: Really? I'm so pleased!

JG: No.

GG: Oh.

JS: Artificial sweeteners are, of course, lab experiments, unnatural substances created in some test tube. Although the evidence is mounting that many are toxic, the jury is still out on exactly what negative effects they have on our bodies. Additionally, even though they don't contain calories, they can still cause insulin levels to spike when you eat them. No artificial sweeteners.

GG: Anything else on the NO list?

JS: Two more things - dairy is one of them.

GG: Ok, I'm outta here. I LOVE CHEESE. That's a deal breaker for me. Grains was bad enough and now cheese?!? Haven't you seen all the happy cows that make the cheese??

JG: Hear us out please.

GG: Ok, but it better be good.

JG: 97% of non-Scandanavians can't process lactose effectively after childhood.

GG: What's lactose? A fancy name for milk?

JS: Close. Lactose is the sugar in dairy products. Most humans don't produce enough lactase, the substance needed to digest lactose, to consume significant quantities of dairy. The result of consuming dairy is poor digestion, bloating, gas, and even pain.

GG: Ok, so no yogurt or milk?

JG: Nope. Yogurt and milk contain lactose.

GG: What about cheese?

JS: It has much less lactose, but it does contain a protein called casein. Unfortunately many humans are sensitive to casein. We recommend that you avoid including cheese in your diet for 30 days. I personally eat a little cheese here and there, but many people react badly to it and don't figure out that cheese is a problem until they go without it for a while. Think of your cheese-free period like a hard-drive reboot with the command key held down.

JG: Geek.

JS: It's not easy being cheesy. There is some good news though. Heavy cream contains almost no lactose, and no casein. It's almost pure fat. Feel free to add some to your coffee, or mashed in your sweet potatoes. Butter contains some small amounts of lactose and casein and is probably ok for most people too. But to be absolutely safe use ghee - clarified butter. It's pure, solid, butterfat with the proteins removed naturally.

GG: What's next?

JG: Seed and vegetable oils and fats. We cover this in lots more depth in the chapter *Fat*, but here's the skinny.

JS: Ba-dum tish.

JG: Take my wife, please. Canola, flax, rapeseed, peanut, sunflower seed, safflower seed, soybean, and corn oils, margarines and spreads are bad news. They are often rancid, or contain too many Omega-6 polyunsaturated fatty acids. When heated or used for cooking, they break down into inflammatory, toxic compounds. They are even inflammatory when consumed cold.

JS: Extra-virgin olive oil is a healthy monounsaturated fat cold, but also breaks down into toxins at cooking temperatures. Coconut oil is a saturated fat that's great for cooking because it stays stable at high temperatures. Avocado oil is also good. Animal fat, like bacon fat, duck fat, or beef tallow, is even better.

GG: How about butter for cooking?

JG: For 90% or so of the population, it's ok. It is technically dairy, as it does contain small amounts of lactose and casein. However, we don't eat nearly the same amounts of butter as we would yogurt or milk - so it's really a question of practicality. Most paleo people are fine eating it in their first 30 days. For a minority of us, the small amounts of lactose and casein ingested in normal servings of butter can be a problem. Those people are better off making or buying ghee. Don't even consider margarines or other vegetable oil concoctions. As we mentioned above, they are full of the unhealthy types of polyunsaturated fatty acids or even trans fats.

GG: Ok, anything else on the NO list?

JS: Just one more. Soy. Aside from being a legume, it's got a few other serious problems.

JG: Here it comes.

GG: I thought soy was good for you?

JG: I saw that coming.

JS: Soy contains phytoestrogens, vegetable versions of the hormone estrogen. Women who eat soy elevate estrogen levels and increase the likelihood of certain cancers. Men get low testosterone, impotence, and man-boobs.

GG: OOOOO!!! REALLY?!??!? I HAVE TO GET ME SOME OF THAT!!!

JG: I know, right? Although some research suggests that phytoestrogens actually regulate hormonal levels instead of raising them, we think the preponderance of evidence disagrees with that view.

JS: There you go. One soybean or a few drops of soy sauce isn't going to make you grow breasts overnight, but we recommend that you drop the soy. Personally, I am not touching the stuff ever again.

JG: It must be the amazing taste of tofu that keeps people coming back for more.

GG: Ok, are we done with the NOs?

JS: YES. And thus it's time to talk about the YES list! Paleo is about HIGH QUALITY FOODS. There's more you need to know! Yeah! Wooo-hoo!!!

JG: Maybe you need a cold shower, bro.

JS: Sorry. I get excited. Number one on the YES list is meat-animal protein. Meat is the most concentrated source of just about every nutrient necessary to humans, including important vitamins, minerals, healthy fats, and essential amino acids. Animals that are fed a proper diet produce far superior meat, of course. As an example, grass-fed beef is preferred over grain fed beef because it has more omega-3 fat, has more beta-carotine, vitamin E, two of the B vitamins, more minerals, and more CLA - a substance that studies have identified as a cancer fighter.

JG: I've got a small beef about labeling. If your beef doesn't say 100% ORGANIC grass-fed beef on the label, then it was probably grain-finished in the last few months and lost most of the nutritional benefit it got from eating grass to begin with.

JS: Right. We recommend that you focus on grass-fed beef, pastured pork, and free-range and organic chicken. Cows that are fed grains on feed lots get sickly and suffer from stomach inflammation. Factory-farmed pork is overly high in omega-6 fats, while pastured is higher in the healthy omega-3. Farmed chickens are often full of hormones and antibiotics, while free-range organic birds make healthy eating.

From an ethical point of view, we believe that it is cruel to raise animals under factory-farm conditions. Humane treatment of meat animals, including refraining from feeding them foods they would otherwise not eat (like grains), is very important to the paleo community for that reason. Jason and I understand that properly raised meat is more expensive and harder to get, but believe us, the health benefits of eating it are huge. It's money well spent. Hit up your local farmers markets or sign up for farm meat-shares and you may be surprised by the reasonable prices.

JG: Don't just focus on expensive cuts of meat, either. Organ meats are even more concentrated in nutrients than muscle meat, and are far less expensive. Don't forget to eat your liver!

GG: What about fish?

JG: Salmon, sardines, and mackerel are the best fish choices because they are highest in healthy omega 3 fat. We will get into this in depth in the chapter called *Fats,* but omega 3 is the kind of polyunsaturated fat we recommend that you eat. Any fish that isn't farm-raised is a good choice. Be careful with tuna, swordfish, or other ocean predators at the top of the food chain. Although these fish are healthy choices naturally, humans have unfortunately polluted the oceans with mercury and other toxic metals that often linger in the meat of these large carnivorous fish.

GG: Does the YES list include shellfish?

JG: Yes. Shrimp, clams, scallops, and mussels are all excellent. Oysters, for example, are full of zinc, which is important to make testosterone which men and women both need. They are also full of vitamins A, B, E, and selenium.

JS: Selenium and zinc also boost testosterone.

JG: All shellfish are just bursting with vitamins and minerals - they are almost as healthy as organ meat. They are superfoods. Eat them often.

GG: Eggs?

JS: Eggs are terrific. Pastured eggs (from chickens that eat insects and a natural diet) are better because they contain more nutrients - you can see it in the dark orange color of the yolks. Also please note: Chickens are not vegetarians. Avoid vegetarian-fed and soy-fed chicken eggs, they have less nutrients.

GG: Everything I've read says I am going to drop dead of heart disease from eating all the meat you recommend. Won't my arteries and veins clog up with cholesterol?

JG: You might drop dead, but it won't be from eating well-raised meat.

JS: Nope. We'll get into this extensively later on, but that very same saturated fat mega-study we mentioned earlier shows pretty conclusively that the saturated fat in well-raised meat doesn't result in increased risk of heart disease.

JG: In fact, the dietary culprit in raising the kind of cholesterol that causes heart disease is processed carbohydrates and refined sugars.

JS: Let's talk about fruits and vegetables.

JG: Almost all fruits and vegetables are fine.

GG: Almost?

JS: Don't go ape with bananas, grapes, apples, and pears because they have lots of sugar. We recommend that you focus on berries, cantaloupe, and other lower sugar fruits. Be careful with dried fruit, because the sugar concentration goes up a lot when they are dried.

Vegetables from the nightshade family, like tomatoes, peppers, and potatoes, can be problematic to those that are sensitive to them, or have autoimmune issues. Avoid eating potato skins because they contain toxic compounds called glycoalkaloids. Remember that sweet potatoes are NOT nightshades, and you can eat them safely, including the skins.

GG: Ha ha, go ape with bananas, you so funny. So I should cut nightshades out for 30 days and then bring them back to see how I do?

JG: Exactly. You're getting the hang of this.

JS: Nuts.

JG: What's wrong?

JS: I mean we need a talk about nuts.

JG: Oh yeah. Well, peanuts are legumes, so they are out.

GG: And they have too much salt on them, right?

JG: Well, in the salt department, your mineral requirements decrease when you eat in a paleo way because absorption is no longer blocked by anti-nutrients in unhealthy foods. You don't need as much sodium in your diet as before because the sodium you eat is better absorbed. However, you're giving up processed and baked goods which are full of excess salt, so you might crave sodium at first. You'll want to add salt to your food to compensate in the first few weeks. Once you adjust, listen to your body and season to taste.

JS: We were talking about nuts, Jason.

JG: Ah. You should be concerned about the oils used to roast nuts. They are usually the bad oils we talk about in the chapter *Fat*. You best bet is raw or dry roasted.

JS: Remember that nuts also contain high quantities of phytic acid, which bind to minerals and prevent their absorption. On the other hand, they contain protein, vitamins B and E, and many important minerals. Some have high levels of healthy omega-3 fat, like walnuts. So nuts are at the top of our *Moderation* list.

JG: The consensus is that a few servings a week of an ounce or two of nuts, or a big spoonful of healthy nut butter, is fine. In particular, a big scoop of almond butter is a great appetite suppressant when you are craving sugars at night. Don't go nuts with the nuts, though. If you overindulge, the drawbacks of the phytic acid outweigh the benefit of the nutrients.

GG: *Can I go now?*

JG: No. We need to talk about gut health to tie this all together. The vast majority of Americans have unhealthy guts - the inevitable result of the grain and legume heavy, highly processed standard American diet. As you know, poor gut health can lead to autoimmune diseases and countless other ailments. When you eat unhealthy foods you systematically damage your gut and undermine your overall health.

GG: *How do you know if your gut is healthy?*

JG: Most people only find out when their gut is unhealthy and they get sick. You can get a stool test if you want to find out for sure.

GG: *Yikes. Stool-tester. Man, I am happy I don't have that job.*

JS: Let's make it simple. The gut is a veritable microbial playground-full of billions of bacteria, both beneficial and harmful. You want to make sure that your gut is populated with enough good bacteria to fight off the bad bacteria so they don't take over down there. To help tilt the balance, we use probiotics - live bacteria in the food we eat.

GG: Yes. But cavemen didn't have probiotics!!!

JS: We are wary of the caveman talk, but in fact they actually did - they got it when they ate dirt. The dirt on their food contained lots of good bacteria which kept their guts healthy.

GG: I ain't eatin' no dirt.

JG: You don't need to. There are lots of ways you can get live bacteria in your diet. Small amounts of kombucha, sauerkraut, kimchee, kefir, and other fermented foods are great sources of bacteria, or you can take supplements if you can get them stored fresh so the bacteria stay alive.

GG: Ok, so gut health is big, I need to make sure I get lots of living bacteria in my intestines, sounds like a lot of fun.

JS: It IS FUN! It's about feeling freaking AMAZING because you are finally at your natural and optimal health level! WOO-HOOO!

JG: Time for Joe's second cold shower of the chapter.

GG: Anything else?

JG: A few last important general principles. Eat large amounts of good paleo food, but eat only when you are hungry and stop eating when you are full. Don't keep shoveling away because something tastes good. If you have gas while eating a clean paleo diet, it's likely because you've eaten too much.

You might find that you only eat once or twice a day. So be it - this is actually a sign of fat adaptation - your body is learning to access fat stores for a steady supply of energy instead of depending on blood glucose. Don't feel obligated to eat three meals a day during regular meal times. We definitely don't encourage grazing by snacking or eating five and six meals a day. This will not promote fat adaptation, and besides, you're not a cow.

Also, it's not necessary to drink gallons of water a day. Drink when you are thirsty, unless you are about to run a marathon - which you probably shouldn't be doing anyway, as we talk about in the chapter *Move*.

JS: Do as much cooking on your stovetop, grill, or oven as you can. Sauté or bake your foods in healthful fats, or grill them generously slathered with coconut oil or ghee. If you steam foods, don't forget to add some fats. We also recommend you cook some of the more difficult to digest vegetables - like broccoli and kale - for a brief period of time before eating them. You'll retain most of the nutrients and improve digestion while you adjust to eating more fresh vegetables.

JG: The best advice we can give you is to start paying attention to how you feel after eating certain things. You'll find very quickly that some foods make you feel great, and others make you feel lousy.

JS: Just listen to your body. You will be able to hear it clearly when you begin to eat in a paleo way.

JG: One more thing. Avoid sugar-filled liquid food. Homemade fruit juices and macerations deliver sugar to the body without the solids and fiber that allow you to digest slowly. No fruit smoothies, no fruit shakes, no fruit purees.

JS: Liquid food can spike insulin just like eating sugar, and of course, that will cause…

JG: DUM DUM DUM…

JS: …excess body fat.

JG: Uh oh, Joe. Trouble.

GG: *Uuuuuhhhhh!!!*

JS: You're out of crackers, right?

JG: He ate them all.

GG: *GRAINS! BRAINS!*

JS: NOT AGAIN!

JG: Luckily I remembered my trusty chainsaw. Hey Grainiak! Over here! Say hello to my little friend! (GRRRRRRRRRRR!)

GG: *GRRRAINS!!! BRRAIIINS!!! AGGGGGGHHHHH!!!!!*

(SPLAT!!)

JG: Ewww. He's got high fructose corn syrup in his veins instead of blood. I need a shower. Oh, well. Want to help me bury his head, Joe?

JS: Ummm…

JG: Didn't think so. At least I didn't ask you to help me shower.

JS: I just threw up in my mouth a little.

CHAPTER FIVE: MOVE

"Everybody, bust a move." ~ MC Hammer

JG: (doing the cabbage patch while rapping) Just bust a move!

JS: Stop that. Please. Right now. For the love of God.

JG: OK, OK! Enough with the drama, it's not like I just force fed you a Big Mac.

JS: I busted out the Hammer quote because this chapter is all about an important part of the paleo lifestyle - exercise and movement.

JG: You know, I saw what you did there. I'm not sure I like it, but I saw it.

JS: It's called subtlety Jason. You should try it sometime.

JG: You're subtle like a brick. You're absolutely right though, Joe. Although the most important part of getting healthy is getting your diet nice and paleoized, it's also vital for optimum health that you move and exercise in the proper way as well.

JS: Yup.

JG: Exercise is the cummerbund on the paleo tuxedo.

JS: Oh boy. That may be the worst metaphor ever. Like really ever.

JG: Would you prefer I said the bow tie? You know, GQ says the bow tie and cummerbund are supposed to match.

JS: I'd prefer you stop screwing around, Mr. Versace, and start talking about exercise.

JG: OK. By the way, I've got someone at the door who'd like to sit in on this chapter and ask us some questions along the way.

JS: What door? This is a book. We are just two-dimensional words on the page, didn't you mention that before?

JG: It's a metaphorical door. If you don't have an imagination, try to rent one. I think they have them at Home Depot in the back with the power tools, available by the hour or by the day.

JS: -_- What-ev.

JG: Anyway, I'd like introduce everyone to Mr. Claudio Cardiovasquez. Welcome, Claudio!

CC: *Hello, Buenos Dias, Obrigado, Ohayo Gozaimasu, Ni Hao, and Bonjour, everyone.*

JS: You're pretty linguistically ambiguous, you know that, Claudio?

CC: *Well, you know, I run all over the world, so I must learn many languages. Also, since I am a construct of your imaginations, my ambiguous nature prevents you both from catching any flak for stereotyping.*

JS: That's very helpful.

CC: *Gracias, Merci, Takk Fyrir, Shukran, Danke, and Beva Kasha.*

JS: It would also be very helpful if you would stop that and stick to English.

CC: *No problemo.*

JG: So let's start by touching on cardiovascular exercise. First, let's define our terms. When we talk about cardio we mean a relatively steady-state exercise session designed to raise your heart rate into a specific beats-per-minute zone, based on age and fitness, and then keep it there for a period of time, generally exceeding fifteen minutes.

In our culture it seems that there's a mystical attachment to steady-state cardiovascular activity, be it running, spinning, hitting the stair climber, zumba, or cardio kickboxing classes, et cetera.

JS: I call it "The Cult of Cardio."

JG: I wish you hadn't, but ok. Anyway…we, as a society, seem to believe that cardio is the cure to all physical ills. Conventional wisdom says that not only does it help you control weight, but it lowers blood pressure, reduces the risk of heart disease, and helps to cope with stress. "Reputable" medical organizations and associations even go so far as to officially recommend at least three days per week of an hour of cardiovascular exercise.

CC: *Oh yes. I agree with all that.*

JG: Somehow I figured you would. Along with our beliefs about cardio, we seem to have pigeonholed other types of exercise as unproductive or even harmful. Lifting heavy weights, for example, is for bodybuilders and steroid-slurping jocks.

JS: You were doing so well, and then you had to slip one in there. Steriod-slurping?

JG: I like alliteration. Sue me. Anyway, according to belief, lifting heavy weights makes you bulky, reduces your flexibility, and makes you speak with an unintelligible Austrian accent.

JS: I'll be back.

JG: I have to admit. That was pretty good.

JS: I live in California, we had to listen to him talk for years.

JG: Good point. So, another set of stigmas has been attached to walking. Apparently, walking is inferior as a means of effective exercise - you only walk if you are too old, overweight, out of shape, or injured to run.

CC: Yes, this is true. The walking, she is useless.

JS: There are no masculine and feminine nouns in English, Claudio.

JG: Stop it, you two. I want to talk about one more important method of exercise and how we view it. It has a number of names but amongst the most common is High Intensity Interval Training, or HIIT for short. These exercise sequences are also known as metcons, or metabolic conditioning. Typically, HIIT involves a circuit of different movements, usually anaerobic, performed in quick succession with little or no rest in between, over a fixed period of time.

JS: Think something like twenty minutes spent performing alternating sets of pushups, pull-ups, jumping jacks, burpees, lunges, and crunches, separated by quick two-minute runs or jump rope sessions, for example.

JG: Exactly. These days, the exercise community has enthusiastically embraced HIIT training, sometimes to the extent that you're supposed to do it until you collapse and throw up. Seven days a week.

Look at the massive proliferation of Crossfit boxes and boot camps dedicated to the proposition that the best way to get fit is to grind yourself into the ground with hours and hours of metcons.

JS: Preferably with someone dressed like Louis Gossett, Jr. from *An Officer and a Gentleman*, screaming obscenities at you all the while.

JG: So there you have it - the present-day exercise paradigm: hours of steady-state cardio good, heavy weightlifting bad, walking useless, and HIIT training healthy, especially if you do it till you puke. Sound about right, Claudio?

CC: *Si. I mean, ja. Sorry. I mean, yes.*

JG: The problem is that this paradigm isn't especially healthy. In fact, it can be unhealthy.

JS: Yep.

JG: To start, steady-state cardio, particularly in the form of distance running, can be quite harmful to humans.

CC: *How can this be?!? Impossible!*

JG: Claudio, let's start at the beginning. First, when you do long distance running, you are putting continuous repetitive stresses on your joints, dramatically increasing the chance of injury.

Second, we've examined numerous scientific studies, beginning with a very thorough 1980 experiment performed in Scandinavian countries. The best science indicates that long-distance running also increases levels of cortisol, a stress-reactive hormone, far more than sprinting, walking or lifting heavy weights. Our bodies react to long distance running in part by secreting cortisol. High cortisol levels can cause the body to retain fat around the midsection while burning lean muscle tissue - a process known as muscular catabolism.

JS: If you look at habitual long distance runners who aren't super-careful with their nutrition, and who forego sufficient weight training, they often retain a ring of unattractive fat around their bellies and are otherwise emaciated in appearance.

JG: Yep. Joe and I were both there, and it's not pretty. Of course, losing lean muscle makes burning fat harder, because lean muscle mass increases your metabolism, so it's doubly destructive. We'll address that later when we talk about the importance of lifting heavy weights, but let's stick with running and cardio for now.

JS: In men long distance running can lower testosterone as well. A recent University of British Columbia study indicated that men who run more than 40 miles per week had substantially lower testosterone levels than men who ran shorter distances or sprinted.

JG: Low testosterone is an ugly deal. It can cause nasty symptoms, including loss of sex drive, depression, and a suppressed immune system.

JS: Low testosterone is just the opposite of paleo.

JG: True.

CC: (flabbergasted) So all this running I've done - all the miles I've covered - all this is BAD for me?

JS: Let's just say you can make better choices.

CC: Like what?

JG: Like sprinting. It's just about the best way to burn fat there is. An important 1994 study entitled *Impact of Exercise Intensity on Body Fatness and Skeletal Muscle Metabolism* showed that participants who sprinted over a 15-week sample period burned NINE TIMES as much fat as those who did aerobic exercise for 20 weeks. Moreover, the sprinters burned less than half the calories of those that did cardio.

CC: How does THAT happen?

JS: It appears that sprinting produces a robust hormonal response that increases fat burning long after the workout is completed. This kind of post-workout metabolic boost doesn't happen after cardio. You don't necessarily have to all-out sprint, either. The key is short intervals of high effort, followed by longer periods of lesser effort or rest. Even 80% effort sprints appear to work perfectly well.

CC: How can running be bad for me? After all, I feel so good when I go on a long run. What about the runner's high?

JG: That runner's high is caused by your body producing endorphins, an amino chain manufactured in the pituitary gland and the hypothalamus. Endorphins act much like opiates - they mask pain and exhaustion and give you a feeling of well being and euphoria. Many scientists believe that the evolutionary purpose of endorphin production is to allow us to survive by encouraging us to keep moving, either after food or while fleeing from a threat, despite the damage we are doing to our bodies.

JS: Also, endorphin production tends to coincide with the point where our bodies run out of glycogen - the starchy sugar we store in our bodies to fuel movement and exercise - and start burning muscle tissue for fuel. Catabolism again.

JG: In the modern world, there's no real reason to exercise to the point where you're damaging your body. Why would you need to, unless you're Joe running from his ex mother-in-law?

JS: Yikes. By the way, Claudio, opiates are drugs, and it's definitely a mixed bag to seek out the production of chemicals to which you may easily become addicted.

CC: Well, you might talk me into sprinting instead of running, but there's no way I'm going to lift heavy weights. I don't want to look like some kind of gorilla in spandex.

JG: The very concept of you in spandex sickens me in a way I cannot accurately describe.

JS: Ditto. The fact is, Claudio, that you probably won't get bulky from lifting heavy weights, but what you WILL do is burn fat and get lean.

CC: How can that possibly be true? The only way to lose fat is cardio! Lots of cardio!

JG: Well, while it's true that cardio can burn calories, it doesn't do a very good job of burning fat. Do you remember the chapter on food where we talked about insulin?

CC: Of course not. I just got here. I was going for a run when you guys were in that chapter.

JG: Okay, we will review. I apologize in advance for getting a bit sciencey. I'll make it as simple as I can.

CC: I love science. That's why I do cardio.

JG: Whatever. One of the most important elements of the body's endocrine system is a hormone called insulin. One of the primary jobs of insulin is to regulate the amount of glucose in the bloodstream, because there's a pretty narrow range of blood glucose level that doesn't result in you keeling over dead. When you eat, the food you consume is digested and then converted to glucose and in turn, the pancreas produces insulin to regulate that glucose. The insulin delivers the glucose to receptors on the cells in your body and feeds it to them as necessary. It takes the excess glucose to the liver, where it is converted to triglycerides and stored as fat. We talked before about insulin resistance and how it leads to fat retention.

CC: My head is spinning.

JS: Must be too much cardio. Anyway, let's get to heavy weightlifting and why it is such a tremendous fat burner.

JG: Sure. Basically, the muscle fibers in our bodies are divided into four types. Some of them, the slow-twitch fibers, are designed to provide relatively small amounts of force over a long period of time. Cardio is one of the types of exercise that uses, or recruits, these slow-twitch fibers.

CC: I often twitch very slowly while running.

JG: Yeah, that's probably the result of brain damage, though.

CC: Huh?

JG: Exactly.

JS: When you lift heavy weights, though, you are using the fast-twitch fibers, which are designed for high levels of force over a short duration. The great part is, though, that you're actually using both the slow-twitch AND the fast-twitch fibers to accomplish the task through a process that scientists call orderly recruitment. Remember that cardio only recruits the slow-twitch fibers.

JG: Exactly, Joe. Now, the neat thing is that when you exercise BOTH types of muscle fibers, you make them ALL more insulin-sensitive. That means that when the insulin comes 'round the old bloodstream, carrying the glucose feed bag and ringing the dinner bell, your muscle cells come running and wolf down the glucose like Snooki pounding appletinis at an open bar.

JS: Great Snooki reference. I forgot you're from Jersey.

JG: I represent. As a result, your muscles grow and there's less excess glucose for the insulin to take to the liver for conversion to fat.

JS: Technically, the existing muscles become more insulin-sensitive as they contract during heavy weightlifting and ALSO heavy weightlifting increases the density of fast-twitch muscle fibers, which are themselves very dense in insulin receptors, so you're benefiting in two ways, fat burning-wise. Even better, your insulin sensitivity persists for up to twenty-four hours after a heavy weight lifting session, just like sprinting, due to your body's hormonal response.

JG: Precisely. The upshot of all this is, if you want to burn fat, lift heavy weights - 80% and above of your maximum effort, in sets of low repetitions, with a bias toward the big lifts: squats, cleans, lunges, presses, and deadlifts. The low repetition point is especially important, because you don't want to break good form due to fatigue. It goes without saying that using strict form protects you from injuring yourself with these heavy weights. It will take time to develop the form to do this type of lifting safely. You may need to hire a professional to help you. Even if you do, it's a worthwhile investment.

JS: As a side benefit, lifting heavy weights helps build bone density, which fights osteoporosis, making this kind of training a great option for older people of both sexes. Keep in mind that "heavy weights" is a relative term. If you are a senior citizen you can still benefit from this type of exercise.

JG: Of course, there are aesthetic benefits. For many years, I was afflicted with a terrible disease.

JS: Do tell.

JG: Yes. A massive deficiency of the most critical nature.

JS: You mean…

JG: Yep. Underdeveloped gluteus maximus. Chronic noassatol disease.

JS: The horror! The horror!

JG: All it took was clean paleo eating and some squats and lunges, and… (turning around and booty-shaking) Take a look! Complete remission!

JS: OMG please point that thing somewhere else. This is book is a no-twerk zone.

JG: Pearls before swine.

JS: Whatev.

JG: I'd also like to mention flexibility at this point.

CC: I'm incredibly flexible. I can touch the tip of my nose with my tongue. See?

JS: Wow. That tongue is just nasty.

JG: As ummm...impressive as that may be, Claudio, that's not the kind of flexibility I'm referring to. I mean the type of flexibility that allows you to exercise effectively without subjecting yourself to possible injury.

CC: Darn. Well, before I go running, I always do a long stretch session. I reach down and touch my toes, I do the hurdler's stretch, I do trunk twists. I do deep knee bends.

JS: Interestingly enough, Claudio, there's quite a bit of research out there that is changing the thinking about stretching. Static stretching prior to exercise, especially before lifting heavy weights, may not be a good idea. Although the muscles lengthen as a result of static stretching, this type of pre-exercise routine can reduce the muscles' ability to move heavy weights. We recommend dynamic stretching prior to weightlifting sessions - a good start is to perform the movement you will do weighted without the weights at first as a warm-up.

After the workout is when static stretching appears to be most beneficial, to avoid excessive soreness.

All that being said, I suspect that's still not what Jason means when he talks about flexibility and moving serious weights around.

JG: If you're going to lift heavy weights, or do any kind of exercise, really, it's important that you build and retain proper flexibility, especially in your ankles, hips, and back. The amount of sitting we do in the modern world - in our cars, at our desks, in front of the TV, whatever - directly compromises the flexibility of these important joints.

JS: Unfortunately things like long-distance running have the same effect.

JG: If you don't have the proper ankle and hip flexibility, it's impossible for you to perform a proper squat, lunge, or other

whole-body, paleo-style exercise with good form. You will end up using secondary muscles and joints and eventually, you will injure yourself.

CC: *I'm flexible! My hips and my ankles are like rubber bands. Just test me!*

JG: **OK, Claudio. Set your feet apart about two fist widths and point them straight ahead in line with your hips.**

CC: *Here you go.*

JG: **Now, without letting your heels come off the ground, drop into a squat without rounding your back. Make sure your butt drops below the level of your knees.**

CC: *!&%*@!*

JG: **Yikes. I see you fell over, and that had to hurt.**

CC: *Ouuuchey!! Ouuuchey!*

JS: Time to call the whaaaaambulance.

CC: *Can you give me a hand here?*

JS: Sure! (applauding) Bravo! Bravissimo!!

JG: **The point is, Claudio, is that many people are unable to perform this simple test of range of motion for the ankle joint, which means they can't do a squat correctly in the gym. Maybe they can push weights around by pointing their feet outward excessively, as a cheat. Maybe their knees collapse inward. Most flaws in form are adaptations for lack of flexibility and will eventually cause injury.**

CC: *OK, so in the flexibility department, I am, how do you say...not so good?*

JG: Not so good.

JS: Claudio, we recommend that you and our readers get some kind of joint flexibility program built into your routine. This is important for everyone but it's especially critical for those who find that they have significantly reduced range of motion. Mobility/Flexibility training only takes a few minutes a day, but it will build a safe foundation for proper exercise.

JG: There are a number of great sources out there to help you learn how to address these issues, but Joe and I are particularly impressed with Dr. Kelly Starrett. His recent book, *Becoming a Supple Leopard,* is a paleo home run. He can help you regain critical flexibility and train yourself to maintain good, healthy spine positions at all times, even during rigorous exercise.

JS: Dr. Starrett is the bomb-diggity.

JG: Bomb-Diggity? You're like a teenage boy, you know that? You have tickets for the Justin Bieber concert next week?

JS: Such an Awesome Display of Pure Manliness. They should put him on the cover of GQ. Love the Beebmeister.

JG: I'll bet you do.

JS: Let's pivot back to lifting heavy things, and why it's so important that we do it.

JG: Roger dodger.

CC: *But what about the bulk? I want to preserve my slim figure, and surely the ladies don't want big manly muscles.*

JS: Claudio, very few people are genetically capable of building big bulky muscles, and an even smaller subset of that group is women, who lack the testosterone to add serious bulk. Male bodybuilders go to incredible dietary efforts to add mass and lift weights in a very different way than we suggest.

JG: A paleo program of weightlifting won't make you bulky. It will equip you with lean, aesthetically pleasing muscle, and that muscle is going to act like a fat-burning suit of armor.

JS: Word.

CC: OK, you guys, you may have convinced me to sprint. You may have talked me into lifting weights. But there's no way you're going to talk me into walking. It's slow. It's boring! Blech! Walking! I don't even walk if I want to get somewhere. Why would I ever want to walk?

JG: Let's start with the reduction in risk of heart attack and coronary disease. Within the last few months, there was an excellent paper published in *The Journal of Arteriosclerosis, Thrombosis and Vascular Biology*. The paper cited data from the landmark Runners and Walkers study. Runners who ran over the sample period reduced the risk of heart and circulatory related illness by 4.5%.

CC: Ha! I told you running was healthy! In your faces, you anti-cardio cretins!

JS: ...but walkers who expended the same amount of energy reduced the risk of the same conditions by 9%.

JG: Booyah. Looks like you got served Claudio.

JS: The benefits for people struggling with high blood sugar levels or who are overweight, or both, are huge. The 2001 Diabetes Prevention Program study showed that overweight people who walked 30 minutes five times per week lost an average of 16 pounds in a year despite making only minor dietary changes. And a 2003 University of Pittsburgh study demonstrated that participants with high blood sugar who undertook the same walking regimen cut their risk of developing type 2 diabetes by half.

JG: Let's also consider the mental side of the equation. We've already discussed how running long distances increases cortisol levels due to stress. A long, slow walk does just the opposite - it's relaxing and promotes serenity and peace. A nice amble through the neighborhood perhaps, listening to classical music on your headphones, is a great restorative.

JS: Of course, when Jason says classical music, he means Britney Spears.

JG: (singing) OOO! Hit me baby one more time...

JS: That's not a bad idea.

CC: I'm totally stunned here. Running is bad. Sprinting, lifting heavy weights, and walking are good. And Jason is the worst singer I've ever heard.

JS: You're much smarter than I originally gave you credit for, Claudio.

JG: I'll just ignore you two haters and move on to the last topic: High Intensity Interval Training, or HIIT. In moderation, HIIT is an excellent piece of the paleo exercise puzzle, but be careful. Too much HIIT can cause catastrophic problems.

CC: You mean like a meteor hitting the earth, resulting in an instantaneous drop in global temperature and the extinction of the human race?

JS: Oh, boy.

JG: Ah, not so much with the meteor, Claudio, but excessive HIIT training can cause similar problems to long distance

running. Although in moderation, HIIT can be a great conditioning tool and fat burner, too many sessions without proper recovery, or sessions that last too long, result in the same stress sequence we discussed earlier: Excessive cortisol, conservation of abdominal fat, and catabolism of the muscle tissue. It can also create hormonal imbalances that result in fatigue, difficulty sleeping, and anxiety.

Some scientists have even proposed the existence of a condition known as adrenal fatigue, a series of systemic hormonal problems brought on by excessive stress (physical, mental, or both) that can have devastating health consequences. Too much of a good thing in the form of excessive HIIT training is said to increase the risk of adrenal fatigue.

JS: This is why we are leery of some Crossfit gyms, boot camps, or other similar programs. Although many of these places prescribe sensible, moderate, HIIT workouts, others push their clients to do five or more HIIT sessions per week, or extend the sessions too long.

JG: Some of the most respected paleo trainers we know, for example, Jason Seib and Sara Fragoso of *Everyday Paleo* and EPLifefit, recommend HIIT sessions of less than twenty minutes of duration, if you are going to do them at all. Speaking for the two of us, Joe and I find that one HIIT session a week is optimal.

Used properly, HIIT will definitely burn fat and it will condition you for cardiovascular effort without actually having to do excessive steady state cardio. Periodically, I will do a distance race or a mud race for fun and as a bonding exercise with some friends, and reasonable HIIT training allows me to run significant distances with relative ease.

We recommend that you listen to your own body, but please, err on the side of caution with HIIT training. Also, if you're doing HIIT, you're going to need to bias your diet a little more toward starchy carbs like sweet potatoes, taro root, parsnips, butternut squash, or turnips. If you try to eat an excessively low-carb diet while performing HIIT training, it's likely you'll bonk – you will run out of energy during the session. You also stand an excellent chance of a hormonal imbalance that will challenge your ability to burn fat and build and maintain muscle.

JS: You have your own little HIIT horror story, don't you, Jason?

JG: I certainly do. I was an early devotee of the Crossfit program when it was just a web-based, solo workout of the day. This was long before the advent of Crossfit boxes and group classes. Some friends of mine told me about this workout method used by elite athletes, members of special forces teams, and law enforcement personnel. The unofficial mascot of this program was a vomiting clown nicknamed Mr. Pukey. Of course, I was hooked.

JS: Sounds fabulous.

JG: For about two years, along with my running, I was cranking out four or five Crossfit workouts of the day - "WODs" in Crossfit-ese - per week. Once a week I would do the infamous Murph WOD, which included hundreds of reps of pushups, pull-ups, and squats, sandwiched between one-mile runs.

JS: How long would that take you?

JG: An hour, or more. I'd get home and I'd lie on my living room rug, sick to my stomach and exhausted.

JS: Just delightful.

JG: Like many people addicted to the gym, I just figured that was the hallmark of a successful workout and the best way to look good and be healthy.

CC: Sounds absolutely reasonable to me.

JG: The problem is, it didn't work. I was exhausted all the time and I slept really badly. I was constantly sore. I had to literally force myself to work out. I didn't look particularly healthy either. My face was pinched and drawn. I had a layer of fat around my waist and although I had definition elsewhere I was starting to look emaciated. I didn't understand what was going on. I just figured I needed to train harder. On top of all that, I was fueling these insane workouts with a diet heavy in grains and low in fat with modest amounts of protein. It was all a recipe for failure.

JS: What does your exercise program look like now?

JG: What do you mean "program"? Should I use one? Like Wii Fit or something?

JS: No, Jason. What does your exercise schedule look like now?

JG: Oh. Why didn't you just ask me that?

JS: I just…ok, never mind. Remind me to edit that out later. Both of us typically do one to two sprint sessions a week, of four to fifteen minutes duration. We lift heavy weights for about half an hour to an hour and a half once a week. It takes that long only because we are careful to rest properly between sets. Jason adds a HIIT session a week, but it's no longer than twenty minutes. We both take long, leisurely walks whenever we have time. We do short periods of flexibility work a few times a week, too.

JG: And that's it. If I'm tired and don't get enough sleep, or if I don't feel well, I don't try to suck it up, and work out anyway. I

take a walk and just do my workout when I feel better. The results have been profound, for both of us.

JS: Exactly. Jason and I both feel great. We're flexible and strong. We don't carry around much body fat and we're layered with lean, healthy muscle. Most importantly although our workouts are rigorous, they leave us feeling energetic and happy, not weak and exhausted.

CC: *I have to agree, you guys look like a million bucks. I figured you both run a hundred miles a week at least.*

JG: I'd rather slow-dance with a warthog Claudio.

JS: So there it is in a nutshell - instead of the old paradigms that didn't work for us (and may not be working for you either) we offer you the kind of paleo program that helped make us average Joes…well, what would you call it Jason?

JG: Ummm…above average?

JS: And you say I have no imagination.

JG: Average-plus? Average with a twist of lime?

JS: Yeah, I'm done with you. Folks, just give it a try.

CC: *And go for a long run every day. Cardio forever! Yeah baby!!*

JG: Can you go to jail for murdering an imaginary character you created?

JS: I don't know, but let's find out. Claudio, now would be a good time to start running. I'm thinking about starting my workout with a few rounds of Cardiovasquez cleans.

CC: *Run away!! Run away!!!*

CHAPTER SIX: PLAY

_____

"When I was a child, I spake as a child, I understood as a child, I thought as a child: but when I became a man, I put away childish things." ~ I Corinthians 13:11

JG: And that's one of the worst ideas that ever came out of what is otherwise a pretty neat book.

JS: You mean *How To Succeed in Emu Farming Without Really Trying*, by Egon Karakov?

JG: No Joe, although I know you keep that one handy on the nightstand for inspiration. I meant the Bible.

JS: That was going to be my second guess.

JG: Of course. Anyway, the implication is that when we reach adulthood, whatever that means, it's time for us to grow up and stop behaving like a kid - to accept adult responsibility and to permanently put away that childish part of ourselves. If you ask me, without getting too incense-burny, new-agey, hemp-oily here, losing touch with our inner child is one of the biggest problems in modern society.

JS: Take your Birkenstocks off at the door before entering the chapter, please, Jason.

JG: Ok then. Maybe you'll agree with me that a major part of living a full paleo lifestyle involves learning - or maybe, RE-LEARNING - what every child knows intuitively.

JS: How to hock a proper lugee?

JG: No Joe. How to play.

JS: I have to say, I like it how you brought it back around to the title of this chapter, and in only about half a page. Also without your usual series of pop culture references and distractions.

JG: Ummm…thanks?

JS: Sure.

JG: At the risk of ruining the recently acquired goodwill, I'd like to bring in another character to chat with us about the subject of play. He's waiting outside.

JS: Tell you what. I will no longer complain about this type of locution IF you stipulate that you are aware that I think referring to two-dimensional imaginary characters that we created as foils to help make our points (and to fatten up the book) as occupying mythical physical space "outside" is ludicrous, juvenile, and otherwise jejune.

JG: I have no idea what you just said.

JS: Just bring him in.

JG: I'd like to introduce Mr. Terrence Trevallieur.

TT: Hey, nice to meet you, listen, I've got exactly twenty-seven minutes put aside for this, I've got a conference call at 2:30 sharp, Donaldson wants those Powerpoints done by close of business, and then I've got to hustle to catch the 7:23 express back home. Wife's got a to-do list for me a yard long.

JS: I'm feeling stressed just listening to you.

TT: Have a cup of coffee. It will relax you.

JG: Thanks for coming in Terrence. We'll do our best to keep things moving.

On a physical level, Joe and I have extensively reviewed the dangers of excessive stress on physical well-being in prior chapters.

JS: We have. You know about cortisol, and what excessive amounts of it can do to you. We let you know about adrenal fatigue and other dangerous hormonal imbalances that are either caused, or aggravated by, excessive stress. You also understand how certain foods can stress your digestive system and lead to all kinds of undesirable results.

JG: Don't misunderstand us - we're not suggesting that it is possible or desirable to completely remove stress from your life. The right types of stress are vital to a healthy human. Exercise, for instance, is just a controlled method used to stress your body in a productive way. The proper application of this stress results in adaptation and growth.

JS: It's incredibly stressful to deal with Jason, for example, but it did result in the *Tao of Paleo*. That's a positive adaptation in my book. Pun intended.

JG: Remember that Joe and I are real people. We have jobs, children, homes, mortgages, and other obligations. If you're an Average Joe, a below Average Joe, or even an Above

Average Joe, you probably face similar challenges, and that isn't gonna change anytime soon. Neither of us is recommending that you move out to the forest, wear a singlet woven out of moss, and spend the rest of your lives communing with woodchucks and french-kissing maple trees.

JS: Really?

JG: I just want to mention that if you french kiss a maple tree, make sure it's consensual.

JS: (sigh)

JG: Dude, have you ever been popped in the chops by an angry maple tree? Not fun. Not fun at all.

JS: Moving on. There's more at stake than the mere physical ramifications of too much stress. It's trite, it's cliche, but it's also true - you only get one life and even if you live to a hundred and three, in the overall scheme of things, it's pretty darn short. You can spend it going ninety miles an hour and working yourself into a ball of emotional shards of glass and barbed wire or you can take the opportunity to stop, look around a little, and enjoy the miraculous experience of being a real live human.

JG: Balls of glass shards and barbed wire are most assuredly not very paleo.

JS: Nope. So we recommend the following one-word paleo prescription against glass shard wire ball-ness: Play.

JG: That's right. Play.

TT: Hold on you guys. I've let you two ramble on for quite a while, wasting my incredibly valuable time. I came here hoping to get something in exchange for my priceless attention and all you have for me is PLAY?? I'm going to call my assistant, maybe she can bump up my afternoon meeting with Gunderson. You guys can go play on the swing set or the teeter-totter or however you want to waste your time. I've got places to go, things to do, and people to see.

JS: Hold on a second there, Terrence. Let me ask you this. What do you do for fun?

TT: Fun?

JS: Yes, fun. Kicks. Jollies. Chuckles. A good time. Fun.

TT: (whispering) Well, you know sometimes, when we've finished all the work for the day, and the rest of the week, in advance, we take Marge Furkenburger's TPS reports - Marge is in charge of the TPS reports you know - we take her reports, and we actually FILE them for her. (giggling) That way when she comes in the next day, she goes to file the TPS reports and they are ALREADY FILED! (laughing) Oh my goodness, that is fun.

JG: Wow, Terrence, you're nothing but a walking, talking party, aren't you, bro?

TT: I KNOW, right?

JS: Terrence what do you do for fun - OUTSIDE of work?

TT: OUTSIDE of WORK? I don't understand those three words when you put them together. Are you speaking ancient Scotch-Romanian or Sanskrit or something?

JG: When you ARE NOT working Terrence, what is it exactly that you do?

TT: (thinking very hard) Ummm…eating? Although I usually do that at my desk, gotta be productive…hmmm…Oh! Got it! Sleeping! Woah, that was a tough one you guys!

JS: The problem is, there are too many people that Jason and I know that are exactly like Terrence here.

JG: Absolutely right. They have no concept of life outside of work and no idea what it means to play.

JS: Jason and I aren't going to tell you how to play, of course…I know what I love to do. I might play this game my daughter invented where she and I hold hands and try to step on the other person's toes. I go on hikes with friends. Sometimes I practice my kung fu forms, and I love traveling.

JG: I'm partial to going to an aikido class or to the yoga studio, or maybe I will go outside and throw the ball around with my son, or play some licks on my Stratocaster. Sometimes the line between play and exercise blurs, depending on what you like to do. Yoga, for example, can be a form of play but it can also be a strenuous workout. If your preferred forms of play resemble exercise, that's fine, but just make sure you adjust your other activity accordingly so as not to risk burnout or fatigue.

JS: Some paleo people are fond of organized systems of play. We hear great things about MovNat, for example, an exercise system designed around teaching humans to move in the way nature intended. MovNat excursions allow participants to enjoy the challenges of moving efficiently outside in a natural environment.

Jason and I are always talking about how much we admire a British chap named Darryl Edwards, who does amazing work with paleo-centric diet and conditioning, but more importantly, trains his clients all around the world to restore the inborn but lost ability to play like a child. If you're fortunate enough to live near Darryl in London, he's terrific. If not, you can look for him when he visits a location near you. He travels extensively doing paleo play-out sessions that are really fun and effectively mask the difficulty and sophisticated programming involved. He can also work with you remotely - check out his blog or his videos on Youtube. Cheerio, pip-pip, stiff upper lip, now there's a sticky wicket, guv'nor. Care for a spotta tea?

JG: Easy there squire. Other paleo folks like parkour, golf, hiking, tennis, basketball, bowling, curling, meditation, ultimate frisbee, orchid breeding, or that cool game that Stallone played in one of the Rambos where you ride around on a horse and try to throw a goat carcass in a circle while other dudes chase you.

JS: It really doesn't matter what you do for fun. The important part is that WHATEVER it is, it needs to be a safe harbor, a calm place to ride out the storm of strife that life can sometimes throw our way, an oasis in midst of the soul-searing desert of the everyday…

JG: (rolling eyes) Cheesy!! Cheese isn't allowed. It's dairy, remember?

JS: It should stop your mind from racing and give you a break from trying to figure out how to solve the problems you're facing. It needs to be a way to disconnect for a little while - to take a break from the stresses that are inevitable in modern life. Active meditation if you will. When you're done, you should feel refreshed and renewed.

JG: Speaking of refreshed and renewed, you're just chomping at the bit to bring it up, aren't you?

JS: Who, me? What could you possibly mean?

JG: You know exactly what I mean. Ok folks, before we get started, just understand that Joe and I don't and won't dictate morality. Everyone has to find their own Tao. We also don't advocate, recommend, or suggest risky behavior.

JS: Borrr-ing. Cut to the chase.

JG: This is one of your favorite topics, so why don't you take it.

JS: Sure. Once you get established on the paleo path, odds are you're going to feel great, both physically and mentally. You're going to have tons more energy-and that means ALL types of energy.

JG: You're really enjoying this, aren't you?

JS: It's part of who we are as human beings. My point is, with all this energy, and the added advantage of all your parts being in better working order, it's likely that you're going to see a dramatic increase in your sex drive.

JG: Can't disagree with you.

JS: Within the bounds of your own moral framework, not to mention common sense, we recommend you take advantage of your body's improved libido. Sex is, after all, a tremendous psychological and physical stress reliever. It's therefore an awesome form of play. And it is very paleo.

JG: No doubt.

JS: We'll be discussing the finer points of the hunka bunka in considerable detail in later chapters.

JG: Oh we will, will we?

JS: Yes. Don't we have a chapter named *Perfecting the Paleo Horizontal Mambo,* or the *Kombucha Sutra*?

JG: No we most certainly do not.

JS: I'm doing the rest of this book under protest.

JG: Duly noted. Can we get back to the subject at hand?

JS: Sure.

JG: **You might spend hours every day trying to get to work, fighting soul-crushing traffic or sweating on a packed commuter train. Maybe you're scrimping and saving to try to make your bills every month. Maybe you hate your boss, but you can't switch jobs. There's probably not much you can do about some of these stressors, but the best way to mitigate them is to find a way to play.**

JS: It may be that you don't have anything in your life that fulfills the need we're talking about. If that's the case, look at it as a great opportunity - a chance to experiment. Try a bunch of different things - things you may have always wanted to try or even things you've never considered - until you find the thing, or if you're lucky, the things, that restore your childish sense of joy. The things that give you back the ability to play. And go have sex. A lot of it.

JG: **Strike that from the record, please.**

JS: Party pooper.

TT: *(softly) Square dancing…?*

JG: **Excuse me?**

TT: *Um…I really, really love to square dance.*

JS: You're kidding, right?

JG: **Hold on, Joe. Terrence, how do you feel when you square dance?**

TT: *(dreamily) The sound of the fiddle - the feel of denim overalls on my skin… Oh man, when I do-si-do, it's as if all the weight of the world is off my shoulders. When I spin my partner and promenande, wow...there's no feeling like it in the world.*

JS: (snorting) Yeah, I'll bet.

JG: Terrence, don't mind him, he's still looking for sympathy between shoe and steak in the dictionary. Obviously without success.

TT: It doesn't matter. No time for square dancing. There's work to be done.

JG: What would happen if you decided to square dance for a few hours a week instead of working so much?

TT: (horrified) What would happen? Then I wouldn't be at work!

JS: And?

TT: You don't understand! I'd miss all that WORK!

JG: Seems to me you already do the work of two people at the office.

TT: (proudly) More like three.

JS: I'll bet that work would survive without you for a few hours a week, and you might even be MORE productive with a little time off for fun. It would have a positive beneficial effect on your hormonal balance, too. Less stress, more energy, leaner waist...

TT: You know, I don't JUST work. I spend time at home too!

JG: We established that. Sleeping.

TT: I also do a lot of work around the house. You know, housework!

JS: I sense a pattern.

JG: Again, Terrence, I imagine that you'd be even BETTER at housework if you just took a little time off to have some fun.

JS: This goes for all of you readers, by the way, not just the psychotically workaholic metaphorical characters we cooked up for the purpose of making our points.

TT: HEY!

JS: Sorry, T. It may be that you feel selfish taking time away from your responsibilities - whether it be at work or at home - to engage in some play. Maybe you feel like you'll lose status or position on the job, or even miss out on a promotion.

JG: Maybe you feel like you'll disappoint your family.

JS: Almost inevitably, we find that those who take time to play are actually more effective at work, and even better family members.

JG: That's true. People who take time out to enjoy the restorative benefits of play become better employees and bosses, better husbands and wives, better fathers and mothers.

JS: To put it simply, they are happier people. And, by the way, more paleo thereby, both on a physical and emotional level. It makes for personal sustainability.

JG: Oh, don't worry, there will be physical benefits. You'll reduce your overall stress level, which alongside a program of proper paleo nutrition, exercise, and sleep with optimize your fat-burning and muscle-building skillz.

JS: I hate that.

JG: Hate what?

JS: When people artificially end words meant to be ended with an "S" with a "Z" instead, in some pathetic attempt to sound hip.

JG: Haterz always be hatin'. Don't be one of the haterz, J-dizzle.

JS: Is there a wall around here that I can bang my head against?

JG: Right over there. Now Terrence, I've got a surprise for you.

TT: Surprise? Oh no, no time for surprises! Ack! We went over on this meeting! Oh no! Disaster! Catastrophe! Armageddon! What about Gunderson? The Powerpoints? Marge Funderburker and the TPS reports?? MY 2:30 CONFERENCE CALL STARTED WITHOUT ME!!!!

JG: Terrr-ence…oh TERRR-ENCE… Look what I've got here! Denim overalls!

TT: (lower lip quivering) Are those…?

JG: Yep. Osh Kosh B'goshes. Double XL, just your size.

TT: But what about work…

JS: Lookie here T! (produces fiddle)

JG: Here, Terry - try on this straw hat, too.

TT: Wow! Fits like a glove!

JG: Hit it Joe!

JS: Hit what? I have no idea how to play the fiddle, Einstein.

JG: This is a book. You can do anything. Like the Matrix.

JS: Do I have to take a blue pill or something?

JG: Dude…

JS: Ok. Right. Fiddle mode…ENGAGE. (begins to play flawless version of *Turkey in the Straw*)

TT: (dancing wildly) YEEEEE-HHAAAAA! This is FUN!

JG: Come on, Terrence! Ace of Diamonds, Jack of Spades, grab your partner, promenade! Throw your partner in the air… ummm…grow a yard of facial hair!

JS: Oh boy do you SUCK at this.

JG: Best I could do on short notice. You know how much square dance calling lessons cost?

JS: Obviously more than you had on hand.

JG: You playing me for a fool again? Don't make me perform violince.

JS: And you had to do that right at the end, didn't you?

CHAPTER SEVEN: SLEEP

"Sleep is the best meditation." ~ Dalai Lama

JG: Homegirl is late.

JS: It's cool, let's start without her.

JG: Ok. Let's talk about the importance of sleep.

JS: I bet everyone reading this knows from her/his own personal experiences how important sleep is.

JG: Right. But what they may not know are all the negative repercussions of not getting enough - it's actually totally alarming when you look at the research. Short sleep is most un-paleo. It can seriously interfere with your journey toward getting healthy. If you don't get enough sleep, you won't have that terrific reserve of energy that comes with the paleo lifestyle. You won't burn fat and add muscle efficiently. You'll also risk some serious long-term health consequences. And after a while you'll start to feel worse than Theon Greyjoy.

Getting proper sleep is absolutely a requirement for living the paleo way, and learning to get enough quality sleep might be one of the toughest parts of your journey.

JS: Most people are probably unfamiliar with all the things that interfere with sleep, all the consequences of not getting it and, most importantly, all that can be done to help improve sleep.

JG: So that's why we are doing this chapter, to fill you in on sleep, and to help you understand where sleep fits in, both in following the paleo template and, eventually, finding your own Tao. Oops. There she is. I'll get the door.

WW: HI! I'M WILMA WIRED!

JG: You're late.

WW: YEAH, SORRY ABOUT THAT JARRON! I HAD TO GO BY PEET'S AND GET SOME OF THEIR AMAZING DELICIOUS KENYA AUCTION LOT BLEND!! MY COFFEE MAKER BROKE THIS MORNING, TOTAL NIGHTMARE!

JG: Peet's?

JS: It's a West Coast thing. You wouldn't understand.

JG: It's cool Wilma. We were just talking about sleep. My name, by the way, is Jason.

WW: GREAT! I LOVE SLEEP! SORRY JARRON! I SEEM TO DO GREAT WITH 4-6 HOURS A NIGHT EVERY NIGHT. I HAVE A ROUTINE I DO BEFORE BED TO HELP ME SLEEP - FIRST I WORKOUT IN THE EVENING, THEN DRINK A GLASS OF WINE, THEN WATCH THE LIVING DEAD OFF MY DVR TO GET MY MIND OFF OF MY BUSY WORK DAY, PLAY ON FACEBOOK FOR 30 MINUTES, THEN POP A MELATONIN AND I SLEEP LIKE A BABY UNTIL MY ALARM GOES OFF! THEN, ONE OR TWO CUPS OF COFFEE LATER, I AM BACK IN THE ZONE!

JS: Uh, well…

JG: **This is going to be interesting.**

WW: *WHAT?!? YOU PREFER TWITTER OVER FACEBOOK?!? OR INSTAGRAM??? OR MAYBE YOU LIKE PINTEREST!! I LOVE PINTEREST!!*

JG: **Sigh. If I may. Every human requires a good solid 7-8 hours of sleep, minimum, every night in order to function properly. So I doubt you're doing great, unless you're actually a lemur, or something. Let's start with your memory. Insufficient sleep negatively affects short-term memory.**

WW: *MY MEMORY IS SPOT ON JARRON!*

JS: Again, his name is Jason.

WW: *YES! JARRON! THAT'S WHAT I SAID JOVE!!*

JS: And long-term sleep deprivation can hurt your long-term memory, too.

JG: **Lack of sleep can have a profound effect on mental health. It can make existing emotional disorders worse, and lead to depression.**

WW: *ALL OF A SUDDEN I FEEL LIKE THERE'S A HOLE IN MY SOUL LEAKING….BUT, YOU KNOW, EVERY WEEK OR SO I CRASH HARD FOR LIKE 12 HOURS, SO IT ALL EVENS OUT I GUESS!*

JS: No, actually it doesn't. Which brings us to general brain function, which encompasses things like coordination, reaction time, and judgement. Just one or two suboptimal sleep nights can impair your normal brain function in these areas.

WW: *OOOOUCH!*

JS: She just walked into a wall. That must have hurt.

JG: Sleeplessness can dull your perceptions by impairing your senses as well.

WW: WHAT DID YOU SAY?!? WHY DOES EVERYONE THINK I'M SCREAMING?!?!

JG: Because you are screaming. That's why we're putting everything you say in caps.

JS: Lack of sleep can even lead to damage on a cellular level and cause systemic inflammation…by systemic inflammation I mean it can cause your organs to swell and become irritated, causing a host of physical problems.

WW: AAAAAAAAAA!!!! I'M REALLLLY IRRITATED!

JS: It appears she has checked that box too.

JG: Lack of sleep can stall fat loss by altering your hormonal balance. For example, the amount of cortisol that your body retains if you don't sleep properly can make it harder to lose fat - yes, losing sleep can easily contribute to a metabolic problem, and of course excess fat retention can cause a whole mess of illnesses.

WW: I'M NOT OVERWEIGHT!

JG: Sorry, didn't mean to suggest you were. Nevertheless, the science is pretty clear - if you don't get adequate sleep, you gain weight, typically in the form of excess body fat. A 2013 University of Colorado study found that a sample group restricted to five hours of sleep per night for just a week gained an average of two pounds. Although their metabolisms actually increased due to the sleeplessness, they chose to eat large amounts of sugary carbs and consumed hundreds of more calories than the control group that got eight hours of sleep.

JS: Another recent study at the University of California Berkeley, published in the journal *Nature Communications,* demonstrated that subjects deprived of sleep show increased activity in a primitive region of the brain called the amygdala, which stimulates cravings, as well as decreased control of the amygdala from the frontal lobe regions that regulate restraint. The sleep-restricted subjects also showed elevated levels of adenosine, a byproduct of our metabolism that can interrupt judgement and higher cognitive function.

JG: The upshot of this study is that the suboptimal sleepers craved more high-calorie carbohydrates and sugary treats and were less able to resist these cravings than the normal sleepers.

JS: Finally, there's the landmark Wisconsin Sleep Cohort study, which followed a group of state employees over the course of many years. This study showed a direct link between sleeplessness and hormonal imbalances that result in added body fat. Subjects who slept less than 8 hours per night also showed higher body mass indices, typically as a result of additional body fat.

We've touched on some of the ways that poor sleeping habits can get in the way of optimal health. Joe, let's mention some of the ways that you can improve the quality of your sleep.

JS: Sure. Biologically, your body is programmed to follow the natural rhythm of the day. Our circadian rhythms are based substantially on the kind of light to which our bodies are exposed. Blue frequencies can increase wakefulness and inhibit deep sleep, and unfortunately, most modern electronics like computers, cellphones, and televisions, emit blue light.

When it is dark you need to stop using electronics in order to sleep soundly. There are even special red-orange glasses you can get to cut out the amount of blue light you absorb after dark to keep it from interfering with your sleep patterns.

WW: HOW DOES BLUE LIGHT AFFECT YOUR ABILITY TO SLEEP?!?

JS: Blue light causes the stress response hormone cortisol to rise. Of course, abnormally elevated cortisol will cause you to retain abdominal fat. It also inhibits your body's ability to generate melatonin naturally. Melatonin is the hormone that helps you wind down to sleep.

Blue light is not the only factor that negatively affects our sleep, but it is one of the biggest culprits in today's electronic-obsessed age.

JG: Here's an interesting factoid - even though the most important factor is to prevent blue light from getting to your eyes, shining blue light on your body can increase your cortisol levels.

WW: SO CUT TO THE CHASE GUYS!! WHAT DO I DO?!?

JS: Stay away from the electronics for a few hours prior to sleeping, even as early as sunset if possible. Get your bedroom, or wherever you go to sleep, as dark as possible. Get out of the habit of falling asleep to the TV or the computer or with your cell phone shining light on your face.

WW: WHAT DO YOU WANT TO DO?? DESTROY MY LIFE?

JS: Nope. More like save it. Jason, let's talk about some of the hormones that are affected by inadequate sleep and the negative effects that can occur when you don't sleep enough.

JG: Well, there's leptin, which regulates your sense of fullness and your metabolism, too. Leptin levels rise during the night to suppress appetite while sleeping. Poor sleep results in a reduction of leptin levels at night and lower leptin levels in

during the day - this, in turn, results in down-regulated insulin sensitivity and an increased craving for carbohydrates.

JS: So poor sleep results in a desire to eat more, and to eat excessive sugary carbs, while at the same time, increasing the likelihood that those carbs are stored as fat. Excessive body fat actually lowers leptin levels AND decreases leptin sensitivity, which can create a vicious cycle.

If the problem is chronic, it can take a long period of normal sleep to restore normal leptin levels and sensitivity. Because normal leptin levels also contribute to a general sense of well being, low leptin levels can also result in depression and anxiety.

WW: MY HEAD IS SPINNING!!

JG: There's also the hormone ghrelin.

WW: GREMLINS?!?

JS: Ghrelin is the counterpart to leptin. It stimulates appetite. When you don't sleep enough, your body responds by producing higher levels of grehlin.

JG: So losing sleep not only makes your sense of fullness/leptin decrease, but your appetite/ghrelin increase. Result: unnatural eating, eating in the middle of the night, and fat gain.

WW: NO FEEDING THE GREMLINS AFTER MIDNIGHT, GOT IT!

JS: It all goes back to evolution, our biochemical programming, and our circadian rhythms.

WW: SIR KADIAN? WHO'S THAT?!? IS HE ON GAME OF THRONES?

JG: Our body comes equipped with several internal 24-hour biochemical clocks. The clocks' rhythms need to be in sync with our environment and the light around us in order for us sleep effectively. Which means when you travel a lot, work night shifts, play video games, or watch TV long after the sun goes down...

JS: You are unwittingly sabotaging your circadian rhythms, negatively affecting your quality of sleep, and causing damage to your body. Evolution doesn't understand that you've got to stay up till 2 a.m. and wake up at 6 a.m. to finish that presentation, or kill the boss on Level 31 of Zombie Zapper.

WW: OK, SO NOT GETTING ENOUGH SLEEP IS REALLY MESSING MY SYSTEM UP. AND TV BEFORE BED IS NOT HELPING...GOT IT. BUT IT'S OK TO DRINK A BEER TO CHILL MYSELF OUT RIGHT? ALCOHOL RELAXES THE BODY, RIGHT?!?

JG: Beer contains gluten, and that's not good at all. But even if you switched to wine...

JS: Or tequila...

JG: Da dum da da da da dum dum, da da da da da da da...

JS: ...alcohol hurts your ability to sleep soundly. Yeah, if you drink enough to lose consciousness, that might work, although that wouldn't be very restorative sleep. Alcohol - like tobacco - increases the cortisol in your body and the quality of sleep you get will suffer as a consequence.

WW: SO NO DRINKING BEFORE BED. I HAVE MORE QUESTIONS ABOUT THIS BLUE LIGHT THINGY. ALL MY ELECTRONICS EMIT BLUE LIGHT?!?

JS: Yep. TV, computer, video gaming console, even your cell phone screen.

JG: There are some fixes. You can install software like F.lux on your computer to make the blue light level that your screen emits go down with the sun. I wish someone would make an app for cell phones to do the same. Hint hint.

WW: OTHER THAN CUTTING BLUE LIGHT AND NOT BOOZING IT UP OR SMOKING, WHAT ELSE CAN BE DONE TO IMPROVE SLEEP?!?

JS: Get as much sunlight as possible while the sun is up. If you supplement with Vitamin D to compensate for inadequate sunlight, take it when the sun is up, in the morning or early in the afternoon.

JG: Also, eat earlier so your stomach isn't full when your head hits the pillow. And don't work out within three hours of bedtime.

WW: BUT WORKING OUT MAKES ME TIRED!!

JS: Listening to you scream makes me tired. Working out is a controlled way of stressing the body and doing it right before bed will prevent your body from relaxing enough afterward to let you get good quality sleep. You want to sleep because you are relaxed, not exhausted and over-stimulated.

JG: And as we said before sleep in a dark room - as dark as possible.

JS: That goes without saying.

JG: Too late.

WW: BUT HOW DO I GET MY MIND OFF MY DAY IF I DON'T WATCH THE LIVING DEAD, OR PLAY ZOMBIE ZAPPER, OR HAVE A GLASS OF CHARDONNAY BEFORE BED??? WINTER IS COMING!!

JS: Read a book by candlelight before you go to bed, or listen to some soothing music. That will distract your mind. The night should be dark, but not full of terrors.

JG: From a nutritional point of view, make sure you are getting lots of taurine, magnesium, zinc, and thiamine in your diet - leafy greens, shellfish and organ meat are great sources, but feel free to supplement if necessary. All of these have been linked to healthy circadian function.

WW: HOW ABOUT MY COFFEE??? I ALWAYS HAVE A NICE CUP OF COFFEE OR SEVEN AFTER DINNER!!

JS: That's not a good idea. Caffeine is a strong stimulant and of course, any stimulant will negatively affect sleep. If you must drink coffee, cut yourself off at 1pm. Seriously.

JG: Another important point: Try to leave work at work as much as possible - both physically and emotionally - sleep in a different room from your computer, and charge your cell phone in a different room overnight so they aren't creating light in your sleep environment. You also don't want to be tempted by those late-night Facebook binges or Candy Crush sessions.

JS: Decide now that you want to improve the quality of your personal life and set limits both on electronics and on stress from work.

WW: I AM SO STRESSED AT THE IDEA OF NO ELECTRONICS, NO COFFEE, NO DRINK, NO WORKOUT, AND ALL THESE NO'S I AM NEVER GONNA SLEEP!!!

JG: It doesn't look like we did her much good, Joe.

JS: Nope.

JG: Any bright ideas?

JS: Too much blue light involved in those.

JG: Horrendous, horrendous joke. You better do something, because she is actually chewing on the curtains now in panic.

WW: *I AM LITERALLY CHEWING ON THE CURTAINS IN PANIC!!*

JG: Yes. I just said that.

JS: Sorry. Well, maybe I do have an idea.

JG: Better make it snappy. She's eyeing the coffee-flavored schnapps over in the liquor cabinet, and I think she just grabbed a *Sweating to the Oldies* DVD.

JS: Hey Wilma!

WW: *WHAT!???!*

JS: Listen up for a minute.

WW: *OK!!!*

JS: Goodnight Moon…Goodnight room…Goodnight moon… Good night cow jumping over the moon…

WW: *WHAT THE HECK ARE YOU TALKING ABOUT JOVE?*

JS: It's Joe. Goodnight light and the red balloon…Goodnight bears…Goodnight chairs…

WW: *JOVE THIS IS ABSOLUTELY NOT GOING TO WORK AT ALL I AM WIDE AWAKE ZZZZZZzzzzzzzz……*

JG: Nice work, Joe. I never would have thought of reading that to her.

JS: Always worked for my kids.

JG: Should we celebrate with a cigar and a nice snifter of that coffee-flavored schnapps?

JS: Are you kidding? It's time to go to sleep!

JG: Ok, ok. Can you read me a story, Jovester?

JS: Ummm…no.

JG: (sigh) Can you at least tell me about the old lady rabbit who is whispering "Hush"? I love the old lady rabbit.

JS: How about I just tell you to hush?!?

JG: Sigh.

CHAPTER EIGHT: SUPPLEMENTS

"The difference between ordinary and extraordinary is that little extra." ~ Jimmy Johnson

JG: Really Joe? Jimmy Johnson? You know I'm a Giants fan. I can't stand that guy.

JS: I know. You're well aware that I enjoy irritating you from time to time.

JG: Duly noted. What's next on our list?

JS: It's time to talk about supplements.

JG: I've been kind of dreading this chapter.

JS: Why?

JG: Because I don't supplement very much myself - I seem to do quite well without any supplements. I know that others swear by them. I find myself in the uncomfortable position of not knowing much about the subject at hand.

JS: Why is that uncomfortable? I assumed you knew a lot about the subject of your hand.

JG: Thanks for the gratuitous auto-eroticism joke. I'm just not sure I can speak intelligently on supplements to our readers.

JS: Don't worry, you aren't alone. I invited someone over to join us in this chapter.

JG: Let me guess, Sylvester Supplemonty?

JS: There's the door. Close, but not quite. Jason, meet Cecilia Supplementarian.

CS: Hi guys!

JG: Psst. Joe. You thinking what I'm thinking?

JS: Yep. Pointy jaw, sharp teeth, long, skinny fingers…looks just like her. Did you drop a house on her sister?

JG: Nope. Why is she staring at me like that?

JS: I think she ummmm…likes you. Hey, Cecilia, what's that you just dropped out of your purse?

CS: Ooops, sorry, that's a bottle of fish oil.

JG: Not the bottle of fish oil. Is that a nine inch butcher knife?

JS: Sure looks like it. And it looks like it's still dripping human blood.

CS: No, it's ummmm…ketchup. And before we go any further, I was acquitted. Not guilty. And the statute of limitations has already expired. Got it?

JG: Psst...JOE! Is that a severed finger wearing a wedding ring hanging on that chain around her neck?

JS: I'm glad you didn't say that too loud Jason, because it might have been awkward.

JG: I'm going out the window if things go south.

JS: Cecilia! I was just about to say that Jason isn't alone when it comes to his views on supplements. Many paleo people don't know much about them, or they believe that we can get all the nutrients we need from food, and only from food.

CS: Well...we don't eat the same foods that we have historically eaten for 99% of our existence as hunter gatherers. For example, we only eat muscle meat - and we don't generally eat organ meat, or other parts of the animal which contain gelatin, which is important for our joints. Hey Jason...how's your organ meat...situation??

JG: Ummm...err... I make bone broth regularly from gelatinous bones, just for that purpose, and I eat liver and other organ meats regularly, so that's not an issue for me.

JS: There are some essential nutrients, like vitamin K2 for example, that you need to get in your diet somehow. If you aren't eating liver or and aren't making bone broth...

CS: Who has time to make bone broth? I work as a traveling salesperson and I barely have time to make my own food at all. So I carry a bag of grass-fed gelatin with me and just add it to my tea once a day, I am big on bagging tea myself, actually. How do YOU feel about tea bagging, Jason, you sexy caveman, you? Come to think of it, I wouldn't mind tasting some of your bone broth...

JG: Uh...Joe...

JS: Just relax. She can smell your fear.

CS: *Sometimes I just eat a spoonful of the gelatin. You know, I'm happy to swallow just about anything that goes in my mouth.*

JS: Yuck.

JG: Yuck.

CS: *Hey, at least I'm certain to get what my body needs that way. I think liver is downright nasty. I tried dressing it up with spices and onions and veggies, but it just tasted like icky funk with spices and onions and veggies on top. So now I take grass-fed liver pills instead.*

JG: Psst…Joe…why do I think she's not talking about animal liver?

CS: *Slander!!! That was never proven!!*

JS: Don't alarm her. Cecilia, liver pills?

CS: *Yeah, they are basically liver, chopped into pill-size pieces. Don't worry, you take them orally. You know, Jason, I like to take things orally.*

JG: Now isn't that extra special?

CS: *And they are inexpensive. I take one every morning. And I also take a couple of grams of fish oil - also in pill form - to get the right ratio of omega-3 to omega-6 fat.*

JG: Aren't you worried that the polyunsaturated fatty acids in the fish oil are rancid? Why not just eat fish?

CS: *Who has time for that? Plus, with all the other toxins that are in fish these days, like mercury in tuna and PSBTs in farm raised fish, who knows if it's even safe to eat fish. Besides, most of the paleo gurus say to take fish oil anyway, even if you are eating fish each week.*

JS: Depends how much.

CS: *They also say the mercury issue in the fish oil is moot because the mercury shows up in the protein of the fish and not in the fat.*

JS: How else do you supplement Cecilia?

CS: *I take 5,000 IUs of vitamin D drops - they are more absorbable than the pills - every day. Because humans are supposed to get vitamin D from the sun, I make sure to only take it during the day.*

JS: Cecilia, you are breaking my heart. Why not just go sit in the sun? Seems like that would be a lot easier and more natural. Jason and I just saw two huge meta-studies on Vitamin D that looked at data from more than a million subjects. It found that while supplementation may be helpful, the best solution is to get about 30 minutes outside in the sun a few times a week.

CS: *Who has time to sit around in the sun? I have work to do and I don't have time to lie around in the sun during the day.*

JG: Geez. That's a lot of supplements to be taking. Let me elaborate for a moment on these Vitamin D studies, conducted by scientists at Harvard, Oxford, and other elite research universities, because they are so significant. As we mentioned above, these two studies looked at the health history over a million people. Subjects with lower levels of Vitamin D were found to have a 35% higher risk of death from heart disease, a 14% higher risk of death from cancer, and higher mortality rates overall. It's pretty clear that good Vitamin D levels are critical to good health. OK, let's move on.

CS: *I also take 500 mg of magnesium every day. I am careful to take magnesium malate, glycinate, or citrate so my body absorbs it properly. Who has time to eat 2.5 cups of spinach every day?*

JS: Ok, well, you have a point there, that's a lot of spinach.

CS: *I bet Jason also has a point. A big one.*

JG: Joe...Joe...she's literally drooling now...there are big gobs of drool running down her chin.

JS: Oh, it's cute. Cecilia, what else is in your supplementary repertoire?

CS: *Well, I know it's important to keep my gut flora healthy, but I think kombucha is nasty, and so is sauerkraut, and I can't do kefir because I don't tolerate dairy, so I take probiotic pills with 4 billion organisms in each. The only problem with that is trying to make sure they the probiotics are stored properly so they maintain their freshness. But I trust my sources.*

JG: Is that all?

CS: *I lift weights so I take 100% egg protein powder. I'm careful to avoid the stuff that says 100% egg but really has a ton of other ingredients and chemicals and flavorings. I get the pure stuff. I used to take whey - but it's dairy protein and I want to be as paleo as I can be, so I now use egg. Whey can be inflammatory for a lot of people.*

JS: Yes, for the dairy-sensitive folks in particular.

CS: *I take a spoonful of creatine and one of L-glutamine every day to help my muscles build faster. My ex-husband used to take selenium, zinc, and NAC, and sunbathe naked to help boost his testosterone levels. One time I went out to him while he was sunbathing and I...*

JS: Yeah that's really very interesting, but let's get back to supplements. Doesn't it bother you that supplements are largely unregulated and can contain almost anything?

CS: *I work closely with experts on the subject to make sure that the brands I buy are the best…Jason, you handsome hunk of grass-fed human, I would love to show you what I mean by working closely…*

JS: Actually, this is the part where Jason and I start talking alone. See, here's the script, and right here it says, "Cecilia makes one more revolting quasi-cannibalistic sexual innuendo bordering on the grossly inappropriate - or exceeding it - guaranteeing that no sane publisher would ever pick this book up, and then leaves Jason and Joe to speak alone." We are obviously past that point. Thank you very much for stopping by Cecilia.

CS: *Hey, wait, Jason, can I get your cell number?*

JG: Yeah, sure. It's seven.

CS: *But that's only one number!*

JG: I've had a cellphone for a really long time. Give me a ring Cecilia, and thanks for coming by. See ya!!

CS: *But…but…*

JS: Hey Cecilia! Is that a Navy ship that just docked out by the pier? It must be, look at all those young guys in sailor suits walking around looking desperate. They look very healthy and quite well-fed, too.

CS: *Oooops! See ya guys! I've got a date with some seamen!!*

JG: And right there Joe, we hit a new low.

JS: Sorry about that bro. At least it's over. I swear she seemed quite normal on the telephone.

JG: So now that the freak show is over, what are we going to recommend to people reading this? She did seem to know her

stuff. At the very least, I learned a lot more about supplements - and sexual harassment - than I knew before.

JS: I think we need to make sure people are getting the essentials in some form or another. The vast majority of people - paleo or not - do not eat a diverse enough menu each week to ensure they are getting everything they need.

JG: So you're on board with something like organ meats, gelatin, 500mg of magnesium, 5,000 IUs of vitamin D, probiotics, and 2-3 grams of fish oil, like Cecilia?

JS: Yes and no. If you are not drinking bone broth regularly, magnesium is a good supplement. Take citrate, glycinate, or malate, like Cecilia said. I would ditch the gelatin for bone broth. I don't care if it is inconvenient, they are not substitutes for one another. Bone broth has lots of minerals in it, aside from magnesium, and there is plenty of evidence that it's superior. We've both heard stories of high-collagen bone broth and physical therapy healing joints in cases where doctors recommended surgery or even total replacement. Like mine.

JG: Yep.

JS: Organ meats are important for sure, because they are the only source of a few essential nutrients like choline. If you really don't like liver and aren't interested in blending it in with ground beef, then sure, go for the grass-fed liver pills, but there are plenty of tasty recipes out there you should try first. I can't go along with Cecilia's advice on D supplements. The jury is out on D supps. It is easy to take too much D, and that can be toxic. Instead, get natural sunlight for half as long as it takes you to get some color on your skin. The darker your skin tone, the more time you need in the sun to get the same amount of D. The meta-studies we mentioned earlier just make the case for getting D the old fashioned way - via good nutrition and the sun.

JG: What about the fish oil?

JS: I would consider half a teaspoon a day of a quality brand of fermented cod liver oil - for example, Green Pasture is an excellent brand – instead. Fermented cod liver oil contains Vitamins D, A, and E, in just the right proportions to have synergistic benefits. Tip of the hat to Chris Masterjohn and his work with fat soluble vitamins. And it's fermented, so it's good for the gut too. We do need to mention that Dr. Chowdhury's meta-study on saturated fat says the jury is still out on fish oil, but it isn't harmful and we think further research will confirm its value.

JG: How about getting the oil - and the omega 3 fats it contains - from eating the fish itself? Dr. Chowdhury's saturated fat meta-study recommends it.

JS: That, too. Although it has many other amazing benefits, the omega-3 in cod liver oil isn't enough by itself. Try to eat a pound of fatty fish each week - for example, that's about one large can of wild salmon, or a few tins of mackerel or sardines. That shouldn't prove overly expensive or inconvenient for anyone. Just add some lemon juice, Bragg's vinegar, sea salt, and/or mustard and eat it right out of the can. It's delicious.

JG: Yum. Agreed. What about probiotics?

JS: Be careful with large amounts of probiotic-dense foods like kombucha and kefir. They are good in small amounts but larger quantities can throw your gut flora out of balance. Ideally, get probiotics from food, but supplement if you have to or if you are intolerant of food-based sources. As Cecilia mentioned, if you need to use supplements, get a quality source of live bacteria.

JG: Was that before or after the bloody butcher knife fell out of her bag and we noticed the mummified finger?

JS: Not quite sure.

JG: Anything else you want to mention on supplements?

JS: Either get a butter oil supplement - again, I recommend Green Pasture, which makes a version blended with fermented cod liver oil - my kids LOVE the cinnamon flavored blend - or if you can tolerate it, eat some raw dairy or grass-fed cheese each week.

JG: Are you actually recommending dairy?

JS: Again: if you can tolerate it, and in small amounts. Other than organ meat and pastured eggs, it is one of the only good sources of vitamin K2, which has tremendous health benefits.

JG: Okay. What about taking multivitamins?

JS: No multivitamins because they almost always contain large doses of folic acid, iron, vitamin E, and/or calcium, all of which can be harmful in excess amounts. Thanks to Chris Kresser for his work in this area.

JG: How about natural testosterone boosters?

JS: You may wish to consider zinc, selenium, and iodine if you don't eat a lot of shellfish. These are all important to get in your diet one way or another, and yes, the first two do boost testosterone levels. Don't supplement selenium if you are already eating lots of shellfish, because some studies suggest that excessive selenium supplementation may have adverse health effects. And there are studies to back up NAC boosting testosterone too - that's N Acetyl Cysteine.

JG: What kind of doses are we talking?

JS: 200 micrograms of selenium daily, 50 milligrams of zinc. As for iodine, take anywhere between 12.5 and 50 milligrams per day, but don't take it at all if you suffer from an autoimmune disease. 600 milligrams of NAC.

JG: Great. Did we want to mention professional advice?

JS: Absolutely. There are a number of skilled experts who specialize in recommending supplements to treat various glandular issues, for example, thyroiditis, adrenal fatigue, et cetera. We would suggest you try this option before you opt for prescription drugs.

JG: Which are, generally speaking, not paleo.

JS: Right.

JG: Because they simply function to blunt or alleviate the symptoms, masking your body's natural signals, and rarely address the underlying cause of the problem. And - serious plagues notwithstanding - people have been thriving for thousands of years without them and have been doing just fine.

JS: Exactly.

JG: I'm still not sure supplementation is right for my Tao, even though I'm starting to get the picture on how they can be helpful to many.

JS: A large chunk of the paleo community would probably agree with you Jason. Again, I have to emphasize that it is ideal to get all the nutrients you need from real food and, like with the cod liver oil, many of the recommended supplements are actually real food in another form. However, if it's not practical or realistic for you to eat a complete menu each week, for whatever reason, then supplement as needed. And do it intelligently.

JG: Let's touch on protein powder and aminos. My understanding is that protein powder, creatine, and L-glutamine don't provide you with anything essential that your body doesn't make or that you can't get from eating real food.

JS: Right. However, a lot of paleo people still supplement with these because they want to build muscle faster and more effectively, and they don't have the time, money, or appetite to ingest the extra food required, or just want to make sure they are getting enough of these muscle-building supps. Just remember to carefully vet the sources of ALL the supplements you choose to take.

JG: Absolutely. If you do use protein powder, just make sure not to get anything full of chemicals and flavorings. Avoid soy-based powder and use egg-based products.

JS: Just another word about boosting testosterone while we're on the subject of supplementing.

JG: Yes. Men's levels naturally decline after a certain age, so for many it may make sense to supplement the way Cecilia's ex did. If you want to feel more youthful and build muscle more easily as you age, you might consider taking some supplements and doing some things that promote higher testosterone levels.

JS: You can try nude sunbathing or going to a tanning salon. Spending intimate time with your girlfriend, boyfriend, or spouse and taking zinc, NAC, and selenium are also helpful. Just remember not to go overboard with the selenium. Just be careful of injections. They are expensive, and they can ruin your body's ability to make testosterone naturally. As - er - aggressive as Cecilia was, she knew a lot about supplements, although perhaps she wasn't going about taking them in the smartest way. She had some good information.

JG: ...for a sexually predatory cannibal.

JS: Maybe next time we should do a conference call with her instead of having her here in person.

JG: As long as she is physically as far away as possible. On Neptune would be perfect. Preferably she should also be wearing a straitjacket.

JS: I think that about wraps it up for supplements.

JG: Wasn't so bad.

JS: Nope.

JG: I just need to figure out how to get Cecilia out of my head.

JS: I'm just glad she wasn't here when you mentioned your head.

JG: (facepalm)

CHAPTER NINE: CARBS

"Give us this day our Daily Bread..." ~ The Lord's Prayer

JS: No thanks.

JG: Yeah, I will also pass on the gluten-packed loaf of intestine-perforating, insulin-spiking, milled insect chow.

JS: Tell us what you really think.

JG: No bread.

JS: Right. However, we do need to talk about a related subject, and that's carbohydrates.

JG: Yep. Carbohydrates are considered a macronutrient, which is a fancy way of saying that it's one of the three types of foods that humans eat the most of, along with protein and fat.

JS: Carbohydrates have gotten mixed reviews in the last few decades, especially since the advent of the Atkins diet.

JG: We're going to take a look at carbohydrates in a paleo context. However, as usual, I've recruited some help.

JS: (slapping forehead) Oh no. Again?

JG: Oh yes. Again.

JS: Very well.

JG: Joe, meet Ms. Claudette Carbonara.

CC: *Buena Sera, Buena Sera! I brought for you a nice plate of some delicious pasta, would you like?*

JS: Why not offer me a nice plate of thumbtacks instead?

CC: *What'a you say?*

JG: I think that he doesn't want the pasta, ma'am.

JS: In *Eat,* we discussed the dangers of eating gluten, which rules out grains like wheat, rye, barley, oats, and corn. Unfortunately, that includes that plate of (shuddering) pasta.

JG: However, remember that the paleo lifestyle isn't the Atkins diet. There are plenty of foods relatively high in carbohydrates that are absolutely paleo, and we are going to encourage you to eat them. Starchy vegetables, for example, like sweet potatoes, parsnips, turnips, and squashes, are excellent sources of carbohydrates. So are lower fructose fruits like berries and cantaloupe.

JS: A carbohydrate is basically a chain made up of carbon, oxygen, and hydrogen. In its simplest form (meaning the shortest chains) the words carbohydrate and sugar are often interchangeable.

JG: Don't be scared of the word sugar. The human body uses the sugar called glucose as a key source of fuel.

CC: Testadura! The body, the main source of fuel is pasta! I eat it every day, and I am full of energy!

JS: I'm sure you are. Let's talk about what happens when you eat carbohydrates, and why we recommend that you eat them. This is a massive oversimplification of a complicated process, but it will do for our purposes.

JG: When you eat carbs, they are digested and converted to glucose and released into the bloodstream. As we've mentioned before...

JS: Or maybe we will mention again in the future...

JG: All of this has happened before. All of this will happen again.

JS: Geek. Galactica references? Really, Jason?

JG: By your command. Anyway, moving on. Your body is designed to regulate blood glucose level within a fairly narrow range. When the glucose from the digested carbs hits the bloodstream, your pancreas produces a hormone called insulin which is designed to take the glucose by the hand and lead it in several possible directions.

JS: Neither glucose molecules or insulin molecules have hands.

JG: They do. Cute little molecular hands with little Mickey Mouse style gloves.

JS: A certain amount of the glucose is converted to a starch called glycogen and stored in the muscles and the liver. The muscle glycogen is isolated and is used for muscular exertion. The liver glycogen is available to the body as necessary, triggered by the release of a hormone called glucagon, which is released when the body senses low blood sugar. Some of the glucose is fed to the cells of your body, or "up-taken." How much depends on insulin sensitivity, which is a fancy way of saying how clearly the cells in your body hear the chemical signals sent by insulin, telling them it's supper time, and also how well they up-take, or absorb, the glucose.

JG: It's all good so far, up until now. The excess glucose is now carried to the liver, where it is converted to triglycerides, and stored...

JS: DUM DUM DUM...

JG: In the FAT cells.

CC: Are you boys saying that I'mma fat??

JS: We would never make such a value judgement.

JG: No way. So clearly the challenge is to have excess sugar from the digestion of carbs NOT get stored as fat. However, if it was a simple matter of avoiding a negative, then the simple answer would be don't eat carbs.

JS: It's like my doctor said when I went and told him it hurt when I moved my arm to the left. He said, "Don't move your arm to the left."

JG: Ba-dum tish.

JS: I'll be here all week. Don't forget to tip your waitress, and be sure to try the veal.

JG: But it's not as simple as "don't eat carbs." We are better with carbohydrates. Although humans can survive without them, and in certain limited cases it makes sense to eat them

in small amounts, as a general statement, carb intake is necessary for optimal health.

JS: If you exercise anaerobically, the source of energy for those workouts is going to come not primarily from fat, but from muscle glycogen and liver glycogen, which comes from the storage of the carbohydrates you eat. Also, if you want your muscles to recover and grow after a workout, your muscle cells need to be fed both amino acids and readily available glucose, the best source of which comes from carbohydrates.

JG: If your workouts are the kind we recommend - short and high intensity, or heavy weight/high effort based, you need that glycogen to fuel your training. That means you need to eat carbs in sufficient quantities 8 -12 hours before your training session.

We also want to re-stock that spent glycogen, and feed the muscles we just trained with lots of glucose and amino acids so that they can grow. When we do paleo-style training like lifting heavy weights or sprinting, we are increasing insulin sensitivity post-workout and our muscle cells are poised to uptake a lot of glucose, so we need to eat carbs shortly AFTER our workout as well.

JS: Most of our bodies aren't metabolically slick enough to sufficiently access fat stores to fuel high-intensity workouts when glycogen is exhausted. So if you aren't sufficiently carbed up-filled with glycogen pre-workout, you will likely run out of energy during your training session. This is known as bonking.

JG: Yes. It is roughly as fun as getting smacked in the face with a frozen halibut.

JS: I've never had that happen to me. I'm adept at dodging seafood.

JG: Not recommended. After the face-slapping comes the part where your body starts to break down muscle tissue for energy, which of course, we want to avoid.

If you fail to eat sufficient carbohydrates AFTER your workout, you won't restore glycogen, setting up an energy deficit for the next time you work out, or even get up to make breakfast, play ball with the kiddies, or walk the dog. You will also fail to feed your muscle cells, which have just been stressed during training and want very badly to snack on some aminos and glucose to recover and multiply.

A post-workout dose of carbs mixed with protein, and the resulting spike of insulin is actually a good biological adaptation. The insulin delivers amino acids from the protein in the meal to the muscle cells along with the glucose, promoting muscle recovery and growth.

JS: Jason made an important point. You don't need to be engaged in formal workouts in order to need carbs for energy. You need carbs in order to fuel relatively routine day-to-day activities that require effort or movement.

JG: The bottom line is: If reasonably active, most of us need to eat carbs, preferably timed to support physical activities properly.

JS: Paleo is not a low *carb* diet, it's low *crap* diet. We don't care so much about the ratio of protein, fats, and carbs, and instead value high quality ingredients. There's a reason that the paleo lifestyle includes certain carbs and not others. Obviously, we exclude carbs such as grains because of the effect of those grains on our digestion.

CC: *Again with the digestion! No one has a problem digesting my pasta!*

JS: Was that noise I heard a few minutes ago a stray car horn, or a lovesick moose?

CC: Just a little bitta da gas.

JG: And that, Claudia, is how you can tell you've eaten something your body doesn't like.

JS: Please note that most of the paleo-friendly carbs we mentioned are kind of like time-release pills. Our body digests them relatively slowly and they don't generate huge blood glucose spikes like eating refined sugar, white bread, or pasta do. Therefore the glucose-insulin reaction is moderated, and because there is less ambient blood glucose, there's less extra to be stored as fat.

JG: In the case of fruit, fructose doesn't spike insulin, although in excessive amounts it does decrease insulin sensitivity, which is undesirable. Thus we recommend relatively low-fructose fruit like berries and cantaloupe.

JS: Because your brain does function best on some glucose, ingestion of moderate carbohydrates support good, healthy brain function, mood, and mental sharpness.

JG: We don't want to give you the impression that we want your body to use carbohydrates converted to free glucose as your only source of energy. In fact, paleo eating is designed to break the body's sole dependence on easy glucose as an energy source. In fact, when we say fat-adapted, what we mean is that your body is adept at splitting apart fat cells through a process called lipolysis and converting them into energy as well as burning glucose, if it is available. Fat adaptation really means metabolic flexibility.

JS: There's another really important reason to eat a moderate amount of carbs, and it has to do with a hormone called leptin.

CC: *I think dere's a lotta dat inna da pasta.*

JS: I think not.

JG: Leptin acts on receptors in the hypothalamus, telling your body that it is full and satiated, and that it doesn't need to eat anymore. When leptin is released, it also speeds up metabolism, facilitates fat-burning and inhibits fat storage, and generates feelings of well-being. Typically, when you have a big meal containing carbohydrates, leptin is released along with insulin.

If you chronically overeat, or are significantly overweight, it's likely that your body has overly high leptin levels, because your hormonal system is trying to stop you from constantly putting too much fuel into the metabolic system.

Unfortunately, the inevitable outcome of this is leptin resistance, or de-sensitivity, where the body stops "hearing" the leptin telling it that it should be full. When you have high leptin levels and leptin resistance, it's too much of a good thing. Your metabolism slows down, you retain and deposit fat, you are always hungry, and you can feel depressed and low.

CC: *Too much of a good thing, like'a too much cavatelli after a big plate'a da ziti?*

JG: Yeah, something like nothing at all like that.

JS: If you don't eat sufficient carbohydrates, something just as bad can happen, and that's low systemic leptin levels. It causes many of the same symptoms as leptin resistance, but it's obviously more prevalent in those who are restricting carbohydrates or calories. The upshot of this is that if you are relatively lean and you don't get enough calories or carbs, your low leptin levels will prevent you from burning fat effectively as your metabolism slows down and you'll lack energy, focus, and mental sharpness.

JG: There are some nasty symptoms correlated to low leptin levels in the science. A 2011 Harvard Medical School/ Massachusetts General Hospital study tied low leptin levels in women of all weights to severe anxiety and depression. It's nothing nice.

JS: The best way to keep leptin at optimal levels is, of course, to avoid calorie restriction or overeating. Paleo people find that eating regular side orders of starchy carbohydrates, particularly pre and post-workout, also helps.

JG: Some of our paleo peers who have set out on their own Tao alternate low carb days with carb "refeeds" - days of higher carbohydrate consumption. They use this strategy in order to optimize their leptin levels for fat burning, amongst other things.

CC: Tell them to call me for'a da refeed! I will make'a the big plate of tortellini! Here, protein boy, you try! Itsa delicious!

JG: Claudette, for the last time, that pasta contains gluten and lectin. It will interfere with my digestion, cause leaky gut and autoimmune disorders, and spike my insulin levels, likely causing my body to retain fat. I'll feel bloated and flatulent and I won't be very happy. And it contains lots of phytic acid which interferes with my body's ability to absorb essential nutrients. Thanks, but no thanks.

CC: I have'a no idea what you'a talking about. This pasta has only tomato sauce, no glue and a no tin!

JS: If what we said above seems overly complex or sciencey, make it simple. Don't worry about the advanced tweaks for now - you can play with your carbohydrate intake once you set out to find your Tao. To start, just follow the template and eat reasonable amounts of fruits and starchy vegetables with your meat and leafy greens - a bit more the night before and just after your workout, a bit less on rest days.

JG: We'd be remiss if we didn't mention that there are people who would benefit from a lower carb regime than what we just talked about. If you are diabetic, for example, or even pre-diabetic, either you do not produce sufficient insulin naturally, or your body is chronically insulin resistant, or both. In this case, a very low carb diet might be for you. And there are many studies which support a very low carb/ketogenic diet to treat Alzheimer's and Parkinson's.

JS: If you are significantly overweight, and you have great deal of fat to lose, it may make sense for you to limit carbs as well until you get closer to your goals. Carbs can be added back as you get leaner and start to exercise more vigorously.

JG: Perhaps you're sedentary, and you don't exercise at all. Joe and I would encourage you to start moving, of course. But in the meantime, again, you might want to keep carb intake moderate-to-low - just high enough to support your new movement.

JS: If you don't fit into any of those categories, however, enjoy a nice sweet potato with some coconut oil, some spaghetti squash, some mashed parsnip or turnip with heavy cream or grass-fed butter, or something along those lines as a side dish for your big helping of animal protein and leafy greens.

CC: Enough is'a enough!

JG: Uh-oh Joe. She looks upset. She looks really mad.

JS: I know. Hey, Claudette, easy! Put that rolling pin away!

CC: Come'a here, you no pasta eating pazzo!

JG: Hang on Joe! Give me a few strands of that linguine!

JS: Hurry up Jay!!! She's swinging that thing around like Yojimbo!

JG: Relax Kurosawa. It is done.

CC: Arghh! Thats'a not fair! Let'a me go!!

JS: Nice Jason! You actually managed to tie her up…with her own pasta!

JG: Live by the cavatelli, die by the cavatelli.

CC: Let'a me go right'a NOW!

JS: I'm thinking that wouldn't be a very good idea.

JG: About as smart as Robb Stark marrying Talisa Maegyr, breaking his promise to marry Walder Frey's daughter.

JS: Dude, I haven't started watching that show yet.

JG: Don't bother, I just spoiled it for you.

CHAPTER TEN: PROTEIN

"I would gladly pay you Tuesday for a hamburger today." ~
J. Wellington Wimpy

JG: This is the hamburger chapter? Yummy.

JS: Ohhh yeah. Especially if it's a big grass-fed burger, with guacamole on top, served between some nice crispy kale leaves.

JG: THAT SOUNDS LIKE A TASTY BURGER. Me, I can't usually eat 'em 'cause my girlfriend's a vegetarian. Which more or less makes me a vegetarian, but I sure love the taste of a good burger.

JS: Nice, Jules. Did you know there's no such verse as Ezekiel 25:17?

JG: Check out the big brain on Joe. Would you like a foot massage?

JS: No.

JG: Back to protein then.

JS: Let's get the wiki stuff out of the way for you sciencey nerd types. Protein is a macronutrient - just like fat and carbohydrates - which means that it's one of the three substances that make up the bulk of the human diet.

JG: Proteins are actually chains of amino acids, strung together with peptide bonds.

JS: Are those the things you buy your kid so they can go to college?

JG: No, those are savings bonds.

JS: The reason Dog the Bounty Hunter chases people?

JG: Bail bonds.

JS: Powder you put on your feet when you're itchy?

JG: Gold Bond.

JS: The British guy who drinks martinis and kills people?

JG: James Bond.

JS: Hmm. The guy with the big alien head who put all that stuff into his body with needles and hit a lot of homers??

JG: Barry Bonds. Listen, it doesn't really matter what peptide bonds are, unless you're planning on passing organic chemistry this semester, ok? I'm just telling you protein is amino acids connected by them. Sheesh.

JS: Ok, Ok. I got it.

JG: You know what comes next.

JS: Yah. The guy waiting outside.

JG: Yep. It's interesting that the Pulp Fiction references came up, though. Let me introduce you to Vincent Vegan.

VV: Did I hear someone mention foot massages?

JS: Yes, but forget it.

VV: Have you seen a used-up palookah named Butch? My boss Marcellus Lettuce wants a word with him.

JG: We haven't seen him. Joe, Vince here is a vegan.

JS: I see.

VV: Yeah, ethically, I can't kill animals, so I don't use them as a food source.

JS: Yet, you do kill people. I mean, you're a hit man, right?

VV: What's your point?

JG: Again, back to protein. It's a vital component of our food, first and foremost because it's what most of our bodies are made of. Our cells are held together by protein, and it is what forms our hair, skin, nails, and organs.

JS: We get protein through the food we eat. In our digestive system, protein gets broken down into its component amino acids and used for a number of tasks. Aminos are ingredients in hormones, they perform cellular signaling functions, they are key components of red blood cells, and they are used for muscle repair and building. Many of the amino acids we need to survive are essential, which means that we can't synthesize them in the body but need to get them via nutrition instead.

VV: I get all the protein I need from beans, nuts, grains, and soy.

JG: The paleo lifestyle is definitely biased toward eating animal protein in order to get the necessary amino acids. It is possible to get sufficient protein through vegetarian sources. However, it's far more difficult, because vegetables, nuts and legumes don't contain the density of protein in animal flesh. Also, with the exception of the pseudo-grain quinoa, single vegetarian sources don't include all the amino acids necessary for the body to survive.

JS: If you try to eat vegetarian sources to meet your protein needs, you're forced to deal with things like gluten, saponins, lectins, and phytates that humans have difficulty digesting. Also, you are forced to eat a very high-carbohydrate diet, since vegetarian foods containing significant protein are almost always high carb. We don't believe that a traditional high-carb diet is optimal or healthy - it often leads to insulin de-sensitivity and excessive weight gain.

JG: As for soy, I wouldn't come within fifty feet of it. Soy is filled with phytoestrogens which can cause severe hormonal problems in men by effecting testosterone and increase the likelihood of cervical cancer in women.

JS: If you're a guy, you don't want man-boobs or performance issues. No need to support Pfizer if you don't have to.

VV: I'm still an A-cup.

JG: Lovely. While we understand and acknowledge the fact that some lovely and intelligent humans reject the consumption of meat on ethical grounds, we paleo types believe that it's entirely appropriate to consume well-raised and healthy animals. As an aside, we'd like to point out that the non-meat eaters who are trying to do a wonderful thing for the planet should bear in mind that 40 times the number of species die out as a result of our practice of farming monoculture grains versus if we devoted our agricultural efforts to raising grass-fed meat and stopped farming grains. Back to our point that humans do much better consuming animal protein.

JS: We're genetically programmed to eat that way, and the science says so. A 2010 study at Arizona State University found that vegetarians that don't get at least 50% of their protein from eggs and dairy sources need to eat 20% more protein from vegetable sources than their meat eating peers to get the same nutritional benefit. This is because vegetable protein just isn't as bioavailable - accessible to the body - as animal protein.

JG: In order to make you healthier, we've made it clear that one of your highest priorities is to rid yourself of some body fat and add some lean muscle. In *Move,* we talked about the methodologies for doing so, and here in *Protein* we want to let you know how important protein is to that process.

JS: Exactly. When you exercise, you are actually stressing your muscles - intentionally breaking them down in hopes that they will rebuild themselves.

JG: We can rebuild them. We have the technology. We can make them bigger. Faster. Stronger...

JS: Oscar Goldman just called. You're needed back in the early seventies.

JG: I'll get my polyester leisure suit from the dry cleaner. Anyway, you've just finished a nasty session of lifting heavy things, and your muscles are insulin-sensitive and looking for supper. Certainly, eating a meal rich in carbs, as we discussed in *Carbs,* isn't a bad idea. It will cause an insulin release which will allow the glucose from the digested carbs to be up-taken into the muscle cells and glycogen stores in the liver and muscles to be restored.

JS: That won't help your muscles repair themselves or get stronger, though.

JG: No sir, it won't. Your muscles are looking for amino acids from protein, which they would like to up-take at the same time they up-take glucose. That's why we recommend a meal with both carbs and lots of protein post-workout, so your muscles can respond to the adaptive stress of working out by getting bigger and stronger. I hate to stereotype, but there aren't many vegan bodybuilders out there.

VV: And I want to be bigger and stronger why?

JS: So you can kill people more effectively for Marcellus Lettuce?

JG: Certainly, to most of us, lean muscle is more aesthetically pleasing than fat, but it's also healthier. Excess adipose tissue is tied to greater likelihood of a whole list of illnesses and diseases.

VV: I've heard that muscle burns more calories than fat.

JS: That's true, but it's a relatively minor issue. According to research from the Pennington Biomedical Center, a pound of fat at rest burns two calories per hour, while a pound of muscle burns six.

JG: Neither of those are big numbers.

VV: So then why do we want to eat protein and work out in order to build bigger and stronger muscles?

JS: Because muscle mass has a huge effect on insulin sensitivity. People who carry lean skeletal muscle are much more insulin-sensitive than those who carry more fat. Remember that the more insulin sensitive you are, the more likely your cells are to uptake glucose, rather than have it transported to the liver and stored in the fat cells as triglycerides. As we've mentioned before…

JG: And we will mention again…

JS: …excess body fat is linked to a host of physical ailments including heart disease and stroke.

JG: We've told you that we'd like your paleo plate to be full of fat, protein and leafy greens, with smaller sides of starchy vegetables and fruit. There are reasons for that over and above the muscle-building issue.

JS: Of the three macronutrients - remember, those are the three main compounds humans eat - protein and fat are the most satiating.

JG: That's right. Protein is going to satisfy your hunger, which means that you're going to be satisfied with less food.

VV: Huh? That doesn't make much sense. You guys have been telling people not to count calories or measure portions, and that calorie restriction is bad, and now you're talking about calorie restriction with less food?

JG: You'll be eating large plates of food for sure, but the satiating effects of protein-dense meals will likely remove the temptation to snack all day on unhealthy foods. As a result, your food intake becomes a self-regulating mechanism. Because you're eating satiating foods, you won't eat too much.

VV: How do you know you're not eating too little then?

JS: Your body will tell you. When you begin to follow the paleo path you will be more in touch with your body and will learn to trust your hunger levels. If you're eating clean paleo, with your plate composed as we suggest, and you still lack energy or you're retaining fat, you need to eat more food, because what you're seeing is a hormonal response to calorie restriction. If you're feeling full of energy, if you're leaning out properly, then you're eating the right amount.

JG: It's self-correcting. After you've spent some time following the template, and you set out to find your own Tao, doubtless you'll experiment with protein intake depending on your individual biology and goals. Some sources, such as paleo guru Robb Wolf...

JS: Bow to your Sensei!! Bow to your Sensei!!

JG: Bowing. Robb Wolf, by the way, is one of the pre-eminent reasons for the progress of the paleo movement, and Joe and I think he's like the paleo Michael Jordan. Anyway, Robb suggests 1 gram of protein per day per pound of bodyweight, others suggest a bit less. That's if you're one of those people who absolutely NEEDS a number, no matter what.

JS: You may be interested in things like bodybuilding or competitive weightlifting, in which case your goal is to build bigger or stronger muscles, respectively. In that case, you're probably going to add protein to your diet and monitor when you eat it carefully to support maximum gains.

JG: If you're looking to be a normal, healthy, active, fit human, however, the template works just fine. Fill your plate with grass-fed ruminant meat like beef or lamb, pastured pork, free-range and non vegetarian-fed organic eggs, wild seafood, and other healthy proteins. Make them the focus of your meals along with leafy green vegetables.

VV: Marcellus Lettuce is a vegan too, you know.

JS: I'm not surprised.

VV: Marcellus says that too much protein is bad for you, that it harms the kidneys and that it can even cause kidney failure. He told me that there are scientific studies that prove it.

JG: Marcellus is wrong.

VV: Last dude who told Marcellus he was wrong got thrown out of a fourth-story window…developed a speech impediment.

JS: Nevertheless. All the studies cited by people like Marcellus with a grudge against diets higher in protein forget to mention one critical fact.

VV: What's that?

JG: The only studies that correlate kidney problems to higher protein diet involve subjects that already suffer from kidney diseases.

JS: That sound you hear is another myth being blown to smithereens by a big 'ol pile of factual dynamite.

JG: Here's a quote from the conclusion of a recent University of Connecticut study by Nancy Rodriguez, Lawrence Armstrong, and William Martin:

"Although excessive protein intake remains a health concern in individuals with pre-existing renal disease, the literature lacks significant research demonstrating a link between protein intake and the initiation or progression of renal disease in healthy individuals."

JS: KA-BOOM!

JG: Yep. But don't take our word for it Vincent. Try it for yourself for 30 days and discover your own paleo Tao.

VV: You guys might be right. Marcellus and I could be completely wrong about protein. You've given me a lot to think about.

JS: Thanks Vincent! That's awfully big of you.

VV: But I don't like having to think about stuff. So I'm going to shoot both of you guys in the face.

JG: Oh no! Just like Marvin!!

VV: There's a little something I like to say right before I shoot someone in the face. Here goes. The path of the righteous man is beset on all sides by the inequities of the animal flesh and the baconry of evil men…

JS: We better do something quick Jason!

VV: Blessed is he who, in the name of soybeans and good kale, shepherds the leeks through the Valley of Darkness…

JG: I'm on it Joe! I'm on it!

VV: And you will know that you should have eaten corn, when I lay my vengeance upon thee…agggggh! What the hell is that!!

JG: The power of rice compels thee! The power of rice compels thee!

JS: Leave it to you to have a cross made entirely of steak stashed away in case of emergency.

JG: Just wait until I start reading from the Book of Revelbacon.

VV: I'm outta here!

JG: Another disaster narrowly averted.

JS: I've never seen a real live vegan exorcism before. Death successfully dodged.

JG: Let's wrap it all up in a bow for you. Protein is a very important part of the paleo lifestyle, and it's necessary to produce and maintain a healthy human. If you want to be a vegan, we respect that choice (although I would say about 25%-35% of the paleo community are former vegetarians or vegans). In any case, you're not likely to die from lack of protein as a result. But you're probably in the wrong book.

JS: Or maybe you should say the wrong movie.

JG: That too.

JS: Still got that cross?

JG: Right here.

JS: (CHOMP!!!)

JG: HEY!!

JS: Sorry Jason. Needed some protein.

JG: Sacrilege. You're going to hell you know.

JS: At least I won't be hungry.

CHAPTER ELEVEN: FAT

———————————

"I guess I don't mind so much being old, as I mind being fat and old."
~ Benjamin Franklin

JS: "Let's talk about fat, bay-bee, let's talk about you and me…"

JG: Plying me with the sublime musical stylings of Salt 'N' Pepa?

JS: Ahhh…no. Just throwing another bone to all those fans who enjoy our pop culture references mixed in with the paleo knowledge we be droppin'.

JG: That WE ARE dropping.

JS: I'm never hanging out with you again after we're done with this book, you know that?

JG: I'm profoundly sad.

JS: Have some fat then. It is, amongst other things, a mood elevator.

JG: Right. So this is the chapter on Fat, I surmise?

JS: Precisely. Fat is another macronutrient, along with protein and carbs. If you forgot what that means, your memory isn't too good. So maybe you need some fat which can help your brain function better.

JG: Let's get the sciencey definition stuff out of the way. A fat molecule, in a nutritional sense, is composed of glycerol bonded to a number of different fatty acids. An oil is just a fat which is typically liquid at room temperature, although there are exceptions.

JS: I suppose it's time for the obligatory introduction of the special guest out in the hall, right?

JG: It's like magic, the way you see things coming. Please meet Mr. Albert Adiposian.

AA: Yo.

JG: Wow, Albert. Great outfit.

AA: It's all from Phat Farm.

JG: How apropos. In a typical display of irony, I do note that you are extremely skinny.

AA: I stay skinny by avoiding eating fats.

JS: Ah. I see. How unfortunate.

AA: We all know that you should eat a low cholesterol diet, low in saturated fats, if you want to stay lean and heart healthy.

JG: Yes, we do all "know" that.

AA: Ok, what's with the "" marks?

JG: Glad you noticed. It's the only way I can convey sarcasm because the readers can't see the smirk on my face. Let me ask you this: Why do you think that a low cholesterol diet that is low in saturated fats is good for you?

AA: Ummm…because everyone is always selling "heart heathy" stuff that is high in grains and low in saturated fat…? Because my heart doctor told me that is how to eat…? Because the American Heart Association says the same thing…?

JS: So you are telling us you know all of this because you rely upon and trust other people who told it to you.

AA: I sure do. I am not a biochemist or a nutritionist.

JG: Nor, obviously, accurately informed.

JS: Is it time to trot out Dr. Chowdhury and his saturated fat meta-study?

JG: Indubitably.

JS: As we mentioned before…

JG: And will surely mention again…

JS: Dr. Rajiv Chowdhury, a cardiovascular epidemiologist from Cambridge University, led an international team that examined eighty saturated fat studies, including over half a million subjects. They then looked at the data from twenty-seven actual randomized controlled trials. The team concluded that people who eat higher levels of saturated fat do not face a higher risk of heart disease or stroke, and that those who eat higher levels of polyunsaturated "heart-healthy" fats do not enjoy a lower risk of the same diseases.

JG: The study did, however, draw a correlation between consuming trans fats and a higher risk of heart disease. More on that later.

AA: If Dr. Chowdhury and his team are right, why were we told to avoid saturated fats for so many years?

JS: Glad you asked. We've got a story to tell you.

AA: Ok, I am all ears.

JG: Let me take you back to the enlightened era of the 1950s. People drove cars with big fins, wore leather jackets, and said "Ayyyyy!" while giving the double thumbs-up sign.

JS: They also hung out at Arnold's Diner and ate cheeseburgers and fries.

JG: Yep. Back in the fifties, there was a scientist by the name of Ancel Keys.

JS: If there is a Sauron of the paleo world, Ancel Keys is he. Anyway, Keys produced a famous study called *The Seven Countries Study* which showed, quite convincingly, that a diet high in saturated fats led to heart disease.

JG: As a result of this study, in 1956 representatives of The American Heart Association appeared on television to inform people that a diet which included large quantities of butter, lard, eggs, and beef would lead to coronary heart disease. This resulted in the American government recommending that people adopt a low-fat diet in order to prevent heart disease.

AA: Sounds like a good reason not to eat saturated fats.

JS: The problem is that Keys started out the study with 21 countries and then just tossed out the results from the 15 countries that didn't fit his hypothesis.

AA: Whoa. Not cool.

JS: It's very cool if you are Ancel Keys and you're interested in proving your theory at any cost…but yeah, not too cool if that's the basis for the modern jihad against saturated fat. Very not cool if you have heart disease and you are under the mistaken assumption that saturated fat is what's killing you. But even despite this, correlation isn't the same as causation.

AA: So you are telling me that saturated fat - animal fat, for example, or coconut oil - is good, and that that I should eat it?

JG: We are telling you that the paleo community believes saturated fat is healthy, and that this belief is supported by thousands of testimonials and also the best science, such as Dr. Chowdhury's saturated fat study. In the testimonial department, in his book *The Paleo Miracle,* Joe has stories of several people who cured their heart disease and got off statins and other drugs in a matter of a couple of months by adopting the paleo lifestyle, which of course, includes increased consumption of saturated fats. But we are also telling you that you should figure it out for yourself - don't take our word for it.

JS: We strongly doubt any doctor in the world would tell you that eating a diet rich in saturated fat for one month will kill you. Go get a thorough physical, complete with blood work and a cardiovascular profile, change your diet for a month, then get tested again. The results will astound you. Just make sure to always demand a VAP test, which is a direct measurement of the LDL. And when the results come back, don't rely on a reading that just looks at the total cholesterol number - it is more important to look at the ratio of LDL, HDL, and triglycerides. Pick up a copy of Jimmy Moore's book *Cholesterol Clarity: What the HDL is wrong with my numbers?* if you need more explanation - for your own knowledge or to educate your physician.

AA: Ok, I'll think about it. Then what causes heart disease? Isn't it cholesterol?

JG: Ok, let's first take a step back and talk about cholesterol - the alleged bad guy.

AA: Alleged?

JG: Is there an echo in here?

JS: Yeah. Cholesterol is absolutely necessary for human life. Cholesterol buildup is just your body's attempt to patch the walls of arteries that are structurally weak.

AA: So you are saying that the cholesterol is only a symptom and not a cause?

JG: Exactamundo.

AA: So then why do doctors prescribe drugs like statins designed to lower cholesterol?

JS: I'll give you one guess.

AA: Ummm…because the drug companies make billions of dollars from manufacturing them, and doctors keep giving them to patients because they don't understand the root cause?

JS: Bingo.

AA: Didn't I read about some famous study that fed a high-cholesterol, animal-fat-rich diet to rabbits? Didn't they die of heart disease?

JG: Yes. But rabbits don't eat meat.

JS: And by the way, if you weren't aware, you are not, in fact, a rabbit.

AA: I feel like an idiot.

JG: Stop feeling like an idiot. Millions of Americans are similarly misinformed, including a large chunk of the medical community. Again, Dr. Chowdhury's study had a lot of interesting things to say about cholesterol.

JS: Basically, total cholesterol levels don't correlate to heart disease risk. Also, it's beneficial to have higher levels of HDL-type cholesterol. Eating saturated fat elevates total and HDL cholesterol.

AA: Doesn't it raise LDL levels too? Isn't that the "bad cholesterol?"

JG: Dr. Chowdhury's study indicated that the only kind of LDL elevated by saturated fat consumption is the "A" type, which is benign. Saturated fat has no effect on levels of the "B" type, which does increase risk of arterial blockage.

AA: Ok, so what raises LDL type B, levels, and you didn't answer my question, what causes heart disease?

JS: In order to answer your question completely, we need to take a step backward and go over the various types of fats. First, let's deal with monounsaturated fats.

AA: Do I have to pay attention to this part? Sounds like high school biology class - BORING!

JG: Another pilgrim just thirsting for knowledge.

JS: I'll make it quick and easy for you, trust me.

AA: Fine. Shoot.

JS: Monounsaturated fat molecules have a single double bond. They are liquid at room temperature and solid when refrigerated.

AA: ZZZzzzzzzz…

JG: You in the back row! Pay attention! Here comes the good part!

JS: Polyunsaturated fats have more than one double bond. They are liquid both at room temperature and when refrigerated. The problem with these fats - and we call them PUFAs (polyunsaturated fatty acids) - is that they are relatively unstable. They can oxidize easily when exposed to light, heat, or air, and they can also change when heated. They tend to break down into free radicals, meaning that the atoms in the molecules can have extra electrons. Free radicals can cause both cell membrane damage and also contribute to plaque buildup on arterial walls.

AA: That doesn't sound good at all.

JG: We would not recommend any of that.

JS: Right. PUFAs are found in abundance in grain products, soybeans, peanuts, and fish oil.

AA: I thought fish oil is good for you…?

JG: You also thought fat was bad for you. You also probably believe in the tooth fairy. Fish oil is good for you. We need to explain further.

AA: There's no tooth fairy?

JS: Let's move on to two subcategories of PUFAs - essential fatty acids. They are so named because the body doesn't manufacture them on its own. The essential fatty acids we are interested in are omega-3 and omega-6 fatty acids.

AA: *There's an omega-6 now? Sheesh, where have I been! I just upgraded to the omega-3 last year.*

JG: **Yeah, omega-6 needs better marketing.**

JS: They are both important for human health. Omega-6 is found in corn, grains, and in grain-fed animals. Omega-3 is found in fish, grass-fed beef, algae, nuts, flaxseed, and chia seeds.

AA: *So we need these PUFAs?*

JG: **In the correct amounts. What is important is the RATIO of omega-3 to omega-6. Anywhere from 1:1 to 1:4 is excellent. Unfortunately the modern American diet produces a ratio of 1:30 or worse. A big part of that is our bias toward grain-feeding our meat animals and our dependence on vegetable oils. Grain-fed ruminants, like cows and lambs, lose almost all their omega-3 fat when they are fed grains, even if it is only for a few months before slaughter. When they are fed grass, what they would otherwise naturally eat, their fat is mostly omega-3. Pastured pigs have high omega-3 levels and low omega-6 levels, but pork from factory farms have astronomically high levels of omega-6 and low levels of omega-3.**

Vegetable oils generally have poor ratios. The omega ratio of corn oil, for example, is something like 1:46.

AA: *Ok, so we need to watch out for PUFAs AND watch out for our omega ratios?*

JS: Yes. Basically, most of us get way too much omega-6 - so we need to try to eliminate foods that have a lot of omega-6 in them. And at the same time, we need to eat more omega-3 foods to help our ratios. Dr. Chowdhury's study correlated the omega-3 found naturally in fish to lower risk of heart disease and stroke.

AA: *But you also mentioned other omega-3 sources like chia and flax, right? So those foods are as good for you as people say they are?*

JS: Unfortunately the research suggests that the omega-3 in flax and chia is not bioavailable to us.

AA: *I have no clue what bioavailable means.*

JG: **It means our bodies can't absorb it. Let me give you an example. One of the goals of eating omega-3 fat is to produce DHA.**

AA: *What does DHA stand for?*

JS: Docosahexaenoic acid.

AA: *Sorry I asked.*

JG: **DHA is really, really important. It's a major structural component of the brain, skin, testicles, cerebral cortex, and retina. Low DHA has been connected to many degenerative diseases and results in poor brain function. When I say that the omega-3 in chia and flax is not bioavailable, I mean that you can eat all the chia and flax that you could possibly tolerate and your DHA levels won't go up at all.**

JS: Consuming animal sources of DHA on the other hand - fish and grass-fed beef - DOES result in DHA levels rising.

AA: *So fish oil IS good then?*

JG: **Well, yes, when you get it from the fish directly, sure. However, if you take fish oil in supplement form, the oils may have gone rancid, and the healthy omega-3s have become not-so-healthy PUFAs. Make sure you vet a good fresh source.**

JS: The best thing to do is eat good, clean, wild-caught fish a couple of times a week - about a pound of fatty fish a week. Good quality fish can be expensive, but when you think about how much money you are saving in potential medical bills, it's a good investment.

JG: Not to mention that eating clean will make you feel freaking amazing.

JS: By fatty fish I mean sardines, mackerel, salmon, and shellfish - they have the highest omega-3 content.

AA: Sardines are nasty and I have no idea what a mackerel is, except that they are sometimes holy. I will stick with the salmon and shellfish.

JG: Let's pivot and touch on saturated fats.

AA: So are saturated fats monounsaturated or PUFAs?

JS: Neither. Saturated fat molecules don't have any double bonds. They are extremely chemically stable and also important components of the human body.

JG: Saturated fat makes up ½ of human cell membrane structure. Consuming it enhances mineral absorption and immune function. It is necessary to process fat-soluble vitamins and to produce the cholesterol necessary for proper body function.

JS: We like saturated fats. They are our friend. We recommend that you eat them.

JG: Lastly, and definitely leastly, there are trans fats.

AA: Trans fats? Those are bad, right?

JS: You are absolutely correct. They are pretty much poison.

JG: They are kind of a Frankenfat.

JS: Yep. Trans fats - hydrogenated fats and oils - were artificially created to give products a longer shelf life.

JG: They are a nasty piece of biochemistry and have been linked to inflammation, atherosclerosis, diabetes, obesity, and immune system disorders. Dr. Chowdhury's study established a link between eating trans fats and elevated risk of heart disease. Trans fats have even been extensively banned in some places.

AA: Ok. Got it. No trans fats. So now that I understand the whole fat spectrum…can we move back to cholesterol and heart disease?

JS: Sure.

AA: Ok, so if I understood you earlier, lowering your overall cholesterol doesn't improve your chances of avoiding heart disease.

JG: Not in and of itself, no.

AA: And that is because cholesterol is the band aid that the body applies to weakened arterial walls.

JS: Yep, amongst other things. Also, higher total cholesterol, HDL, and LDL-A levels don't correlate to risk of heart disease.

AA: Well, what causes the artery walls to weaken the first place?

JS: The short answer, and the most important factor, is oxidation.

AA: You used that word before when we talked about PUFAs. What the heck does it mean?

JG: Well, technically it means a chemical change resulting from exposing something to oxygen. Like when metal oxidizes and turns to rust.

AA: So that's going on in your heart?!?

JS: Well, not exactly. Oxidation occurs when certain types of cholesterol - mostly the LDL-B - reacts with free radicals.

AA: That's the second time you've mentioned free radicals. Shouldn't they do a better job of keeping those radicals imprisoned??

JG: Oh boy. Here we go.

JS: Let me back up a bit. So there's that stuff called low density lipoprotein cholesterol type B, that's LDL-B, or what we'll call the bad cholesterol - combines with free radicals, then it oxidizes and causes heart and blood vessel tissue damage.

AA: What are free radicals you keep talking about?

JG: Free radicals are atoms or groups of atoms with an odd (unpaired) number of electrons and can be formed when oxygen interacts with certain molecules.

AA: This isn't helping at all.

JS: Ok, lets make it simpler. First, you need to stop eating trans fats - those chemical Frankenfats we talked about - because they are a chief culprit in this heart-damaging scenario. Don't put anything in your mouth that is hydrogenized or partially hydrogenated, because those are trans fats. You want to eat lots of anti-oxidants - lots of them in veggies and fruits, nuts, olive oil, and even dark chocolate, for example - to counteract the effect of trans fats and free radicals as much as possible.

JG: You'd also be wise to avoid eating some of those PUFAs we discussed earlier. They can also easily oxidize. Seed and vegetable oils like canola, grapeseed, sunflower, peanut, and soy oils are good examples of PUFAs to avoid. They easily go rancid as well, which only increases the danger of eating them. Also, avoid fish oil supplements unless you are sure they are fresh and haven't gone rancid - when that happens, the healthy omega-3s turn into omega-6s and can also oxidize. Generally, omega-3s consumed directly from animal sources are more stable and don't oxidize or turn rancid.

AA: Ok, so I understand that oxidation, brought on by the consumption of unhealthy fats, is one cause of heart disease. Anything else?

JS: Yep. Inflammation also contributes to heart disease.

AA: You mean like swelling?

JS: Yes, in the sense of internal, systemic inflammation in your body.

AA: What causes this type of inflammation?

JG: Eating processed sugars, processed carbs, excessive omega-6 PUFAs, trans fats, and grains. Levels of LDL-B, the bad cholesterol, rise in your body the more you eat these things in response to this type of systemic inflammation.

AA: So we finally get to the answer to the question I was asking all along. Eating trans fats, PUFAs, processed sugars, processed carbs, and grains can cause heart disease?

JS: Bingo.

AA: I thought that heart disease was hereditary.

JS: It is - in the sense that there's a hereditary component of susceptibility. The level of inflammatory response to eating trans fats, sugars, processed carbs, and grains is hereditary. We have a genetic level of response to these foods that varies based on heredity. But whether or not the genetic potential is ultimately expressed depends on, in large part, what you eat.

AA: *So this all just confirms exactly what I believed was true. If fats are so dangerous, then I shouldn't eat them. Yay! Adiposian for the win!*

JG: **Hold your horses.**

JS: That's not what we meant at all. Certainly there are types of fat that are not healthy to eat, like trans fats and excessive amounts of omega-6 PUFAs. However, there are a number of fats that are very healthy, and you need to eat them.

AA: *So what fats are good? And why are they good?*

JG: **We recommend saturated fats, like those found in animal flesh, and those found in stable oils like coconut oil, avocado oil, and ghee. Certain monounsaturated fats are good too, like olive oil, as long as they are consumed unheated. You should also consume the omega-3 polyunsaturated fats directly, by eating fish, certain nuts, and properly raised animals.**

AA: *But saturated fat is terrible! Didn't that guy Ancel and Gretel say so, right before he put the witch in the oven and cooked her to death?*

JS: Ancel Keys. Yeah, but remember, that study was a complete sham. And it was totally wrong.

JG: **Yep, in fact, even before Dr. Chowdhury's saturated fat meta-analysis was published in *Annals of Internal Medicine*, there was a landmark analysis of research on saturated fat published in the *American Journal of Clinical Nutrition* in 2010.**

This analysis looked at 21 studies, and those studies tracked over 350,000 people. Do you know what that analysis found?

AA: That Albert Adiposian is the most awesome dude ever?

JS: That there was insufficient evidence to link saturated fat consumption to heart disease or stroke.

JG: This was hot on the heels of a 2006 Women's Health Initiative study that found that reducing saturated fat failed to reduce the rate of heart disease.

JS: The truth is that the whole heart disease from saturated fat argument isn't backed by scientific evidence. There is a correlation between high LDL-B levels and heart disease, but as we mentioned before, eating saturated fats doesn't raise LDL. In fact, it can lower it, and raise levels of the good HDL cholesterol. It can also reduce levels of lipoprotein (a), which is a key marker for heart disease.

AA: Wow. Anything else I need to know about fats, besides that eating the right ones don't cause heart disease?

JG: Yes. Eating fats doesn't make you fat.

JS: In fact, eating the right types of fat (saturated fats, omega-3 polyunsaturated fats from good sources, and unheated monounsaturated fats) will promote overall general health. Consuming fatty cuts of meat and cooking in coconut oil, ghee, and unheated olive oil are good for you in many other ways besides heart health. Fat helps brain and lung function and it is a natural mood elevator. Fat helps keep your liver healthy and aids in tuning your nervous system.

In a dietary sense fat is a high satiety macronutrient, like protein, and helps satisfy your appetite, preventing you from over eating.

Remember it's intake of grains, sugary carbs, and other processed foods that leads to body fat retention, not the consumption of healthy fats.

AA: So you want me to eat fat.

JG: Yes, the right kinds of fats. In significant quantities. We want you to cook with them, too, and add them to food for additional flavor as well.

AA: You want me to eat meat as well, to get more of that fat.

JS: Grass-fed and pastured meat, yes. And eggs, too. And fatty seafood.

AA: And eating all this fat won't make me fat. It won't give me heart disease, strokes, or anything.

JG: Nope.

AA: And what was it you said about eating certain oils, like avocado, unheated olive oil and…

JS: Coconut oil.

AA: Yeah, I just saw a can labeled "Coconut Oil" over there! Can I taste some?

JG: Wait. No. Don't. Stop.

AA: MMMMM! Delicious!!! You guys were right. It's absolutely scrumptious!! I feel great!!!

JG: Uh oh. Too late.

JS: What did you do now?

JG: Albert, if you had read the label on other side of the can, it says "Experimental! Dangerous!! Do Not Consume!!"

AA: What's happening to me?

JS: You appear to be inflating, kind of like a hot air balloon. What's in the can, Jason?

JG: Oh, just a little experiment of mine. It's highly concentrated coconut oil, I'm trying to develop a formula that will lower LDL-B cholesterol with just one teaspoon a week. There are still some bugs to work out.

AA: AAAAAAGHH!

JS: I can see that. Albert appears to have blown up to the size of a human beach ball. And he's turned brown and sprouted hairs like…

JG: A coconut. There isn't much time either.

JS: Until?

JG: Until he bursts, spraying coconut oil all over our nice clean book. Don't worry, though.

JS: What's with that little harmonica you just blew?

JG: I'm calling for help.

JS: Who are all the fat little midgets??

JG: PUFA-Looofas. They will take him to the cracking room, and hopefully de-oil him before he bursts.

JS: They are singing a little song as they roll him away!

JG: Yeah, they won't work unless they get to sing their little songs.

JS: Strong union.

JG: Yep. Let's listen:

PUFA-Looofah, looofity do…
Don't avoid fat or you're gonna be screwed,

It's good for your brain and it helps to you see,
to be good in bed and to easily pee,

Fat is your friend, so eat a whole slew,
like the PUFA-Looofahs loofity do!

JS: Catchy.

JG: No doubt.

JS: Is he going to be ok?

JG: Who knows? Do you really care?

JS: Nah. Not really.

JG: Me neither.

CHAPTER TWELVE: BREATHE

"The perfect is the enemy of the good." ~ Voltaire

JG: Why ya gotta go and make things so complicated...

JS: Oh no. Please do not do that. Do not sing Avril Lavigne. Ever, ever. This grass-fed burger I just ate was very delicious and I don't want to end up projectile vomiting it all over you.

JG: Charming. What's on our agenda for the day?

JS: You know, you and I - we've talked a lot about the best way to screw up a good, simple idea, like, for instance, finding your paleo Tao.

JG: Yeah. Getting wrapped up in the small stuff. Making something basic and natural way too complicated. Trying for perfect instead of being happy with good.

JS: Exactly. Which is why I sent a messenger pigeon down to Peru.

JG: Peru? Dude, you didn't. She's a myth - a legend to scare paleo children who don't want to eat their broiled liver. She's like the paleo chupacabra.

JS: She is not a myth.

JG: What??

JS: In fact, she's here. Waiting out in the hallway.

JG: Wow. Did she ride a llama up here or something?

JS: It was an alpaca, actually.

JG: Unreal. I can't believe she actually exists, let alone that she's here. This should be interesting.

JS: Yep. Without further ado…Paula Paleoista! She has been paleo since the day she was born. Her parents were paleo, and their parents before that, and so on, back to the actual Paleolithic age.

JG: Wow. I can only imagine the profound levels of paleo wisdom she has acquired.

JS: Undoubtedly. Paula! You can come in now!!

JG: She's not coming in.

JS: Ok, let me go grab her, be right back.

…

JG: What took you guys so long?

JS: I found her outside lecturing a rabbit on what type of clover it should eat in order to form optimal levels of omega-3 fats.

PP: *Pleased to meet you two! I am Paula Paleoista!*

JG: **Nice to meet you Paula. Is that a fur bikini you're wearing?**

PP: *Yes, I stalked, killed, and skinned the antelope myself.*

JG: **It smells interesting too.**

PP: *I tanned it with my own urine, just like our ancestors did.*

JG: **Isn't that just lovely?**

JS: The reason we have Paula here is to get her take on this paleo stuff, given her wisdom and experience. She's a veritable high Priestess of Paleosity.

PP: *On the way here from Peru - by the way, I tamed a wild alpaca because I think flying isn't paleo at all, just the damage done to the environment by burning fossil fuels, all the plastics used in the aircraft seats, the carcinogens in the food...*

JG: **You live in Peru?!?**

PP: *Yeah. I live in the jungle down there. Everything's totally paleo. I built a paleolithic cave dwelling, I can stalk and kill all my own food without anyone giving me grief about it, and there's no question about the quality vegetables and fruits I eat because I forage them myself. Anyway, I got into this big debate with two guys on the way. Can you believe they were riding HORSES? No one rode horses in the Paleolithic!!*

JS: Sinners.

PP: *Anyway, one of these guys insisted that cashews were legumes because they grow with the seed stemming from the cashew apple, and because the cashew plant has several seeds that eventually split open on their own. The other dude kept saying that cashews were drupes because they develop first on the cashew tree and are surrounded by a double shell containing an allergenic phenolic resin called anacardic acid, a potent skin irritant chemically related to the more well-known allergenic oil urushiol which is also a toxin found in the related poison ivy.*

JS: How did you manage to hold your tongue?

PP: It was such an infuriating conversation, because of course, they were both wrong. They went against everything my family and I have been practicing for thousands of years of True Paleo, what with their Neolithic ways. I actually lost a little sleep over it. They are so not paleo. They are anti-paleo. They must be assimilated or destroyed.

JG: Wow.

JS: Yeah. Wow.

PP: So when I got into town, I went to a supposedly paleo cafe to get something to eat, because I couldn't stalk any game. Can you believe they offered me a glass of orange juice! ORANGE JUICE! NOT AN ORANGE BUT ORANGE JUICE! Man, that was crazy. HELLO INSULIN SPIKE!! I almost put on a pound of fat around my midsection just because they MENTIONED fruit juice to me.

JG: Ummmm…

JS: Yikes.

PP: Anyway, do either of you know what time it is? I haven't been able to tell the time since I got here because the stars are all different, and I take my probiotics precisely at six twenty-two every evening.

JG: Let me look at my watch… it's 6:00 p.m.

PP: You wear a watch!?!? With a battery?!? Don't you know about the electromagnetic field coming out of that thing? And you wear it after dark?!? Do you know what electromagnetic radiation does to your natural cortisol levels?!? OMG how do you survive???!?? Blue light!!! Blue light!!! Emergency!!! Emergency!!!

JG: Ummm…hey Joe…

JS: Yeah. Ok, so let's get back on topic here…

PP: Then there was the lady outside in your waiting room…

JG: We have a waiting room now?? With a receptionist???

JS: Yeah, I made a few little upgrades…

JG: Before we sold a single copy of the book? What's next, Tammy Faye, matching Rolexes??

PP: …anyway, the lady, she offered me some natural tea - which sounded great - until I heard the whirring noise coming from the kitchen. I went in to confirm my worst nightmare - she was heating up the water in a microwave oven!!!

JG: Joe?? We have a kitchen, too? And a microwave???

JS: Yeah, the local fire codes don't allow her to burn wood and leaves inside.

PP: Have you ever watered plants with microwaved water? THEY DIE. I think she was secretly trying to kill me or something.

JG: We should have her killed. Or arrested. Or stomped to death by an alpaca.

PP: And the tea was in a BAG!! I mean, she didn't even go out and gather leaves and bark herself! Who knows what was in that tea??!?

JS: Who indeed.

PP: I must say I'm used to this kind of treatment. I think because I choose not to wash myself in chemicals and fluoridated water every day, people don't seem to like me very much. Speaking of which, do you know where the nearest lake is so I can take a bath? It's got to have the correct PH levels by the way - not too alkaline or acidic please!

JG: I...ummm...don't know of any...local lakes...that allow... ummm...bathing...

JS: You know what Paula? I think we are done for today. I appreciate the fact that you have come so far, and I think you have already told us everything we need to know.

PP: I haven't even talked about the evils of tampons yet!!!

JS: I will send you some freshly killed capybara as promised, just send me a carrier pigeon and let me know what hotel you are staying behind. Let me show you out.

PP: But the tampons!!

JS: Jason and I will make sure not to use them. Take care, bye-bye now.

JG: I think you could have made your point with a little more subtlety.

JS: Maybe. But there's an important point to be made. There's danger in being paleo in the modern world...in being part of a minority movement that doesn't accept contemporary mainstream conventional wisdom on health, nutrition, and medicine.

JG: You mean because the distinction between science and fantasy is so fine?

JS: No. I actually think there is at least a grain of legitimacy in everything Paula said.

JG: She would spontaneously combust if she heard you say the word "grain."

JS: What I'm trying to say is that there is a potential to go too far with this stuff. When you start to adopt the paleo template and it works for you, it's important to retain your sense of tolerance. In terms of how you relate to others, be kind and generous. Don't become a zealot. Don't start interpreting other people's acts of kindness as ignorance, or even malice. If someone offers you a cookie they baked, it's okay to say "No, but thank you for thinking of me" and not, "Are you trying to kill me?!?" Don't judge others in how they pursue their Tao either. Acting all dogmatic will just reduce the appeal of the paleo way for anyone considering it.

JG: Remember also that while we start with a basic template, *The Tao of Paleo* you find is going to be a personal Tao. Yours won't be exactly like anyone else's. Accept that others will probably have a different take on paleo, or even other approaches to health, like vegetarianism.

JS: You're going to feel great…but before you take the plunge, remember that you need to keep your perspective on all of this. Go ahead and feel born again - feel like you want to change the world. Don't, however, go all righteous and turn into a hardcore judgmental paleo freak.

JG: And do write books to help people?

JS: By all means, if you are as cool as we are.

JG: We are pretty cool. Paula, on the other hand…

JS: While she was talking I was entertaining the idea of asking her if potatoes were paleo, but I thought her head might explode like those guys from Scanners.

JG: The key thing I took from Paula's visit was how important it is to live and let live. There are many different Taos. Anyone practicing paleo in any form can use your support far more than they can use your scorn.

JS: Profound, dude. Remember the name of the book? This is about finding YOUR own Tao and respecting the Tao that others want to walk.

JG: Yep, and Paula was probably the best example of the worst way to do it.

JS: Lose the dogma. Carrying around guilt or stress about something that is supposed to make you healthy is…

JG: Unhealthy.

JS: Disco.

JG: Pulp Fiction reference again Uma?

JS: Yep.

JG: Got it. You're weird.

JS: About time you noticed.

JG: Let's bring this back around. Remember that you're going to start your paleo journey by following a template, and at first we'd like to help you keep it simple for your own sanity. It's pretty important to follow our guidelines on the big issues, but don't sweat the small stuff. Don't feel like you need to adopt every little tenet of the paleo path that others think is important.

JS: There's no need to jump head first into making kombucha on day one - or your own toothpaste for that matter. There's also no need to let all those loud voices squabbling about the finer points worry you.

If we are to succeed as a movement and actually make the world healthier and happier, we need to be inclusive, not divisive. We need to stand united with our brethren, even if they happen to add soy sauce to their salad once a week or snack on spoonfuls of peanut butter.

JG: We about ready to wrap this one up?

JS: Yeah, except we wanted to mention cheating.

JG: Right. Paula might have a conniption if she found out someone slipped some cane sugar into her sweet potatoes, but you don't need to sweat the small stuff. Don't beat yourself up for falling off the wagon. And it's not cheating. It's a choice. Guilt and food should never be associated with one another.

JS: Excellent point Jason. Nobody is perfect. Don't agonize over eating a cookie every other day, or even if you go on a major binge. It's not easy to change your life. If you had a plan and it didn't work perfectly, for whatever reason, set new goals, get back on track, and stick to it as best you can. Repeat as many times as it takes. You will succeed.

JG: Just remember this - we are trying to change the world into a healthier place. We are at the forefront of a peaceful, healing, real-food revolution. We are HEROES in that sense, and our efforts are for a larger cause - beyond simply becoming healthier and happier.

JS: And guess what? The second you picked up this book, you joined forces with us, and with The Paleo Movement. You're a hero too.

JG: Wonder Twins powers activated. Congratulations. And welcome aboard. We're proud of you already.

JS: Just don't be a jerk like Paula.

JG: Agreed.

JS: And don't wear urine-soaked fur bikinis.

JG: Yeah, that too.

CHAPTER THIRTEEN: FEEL

"A Jedi can feel the Force flowing through him." ~ Obi Wan Kenobi

JG: Ok Joe, so first *Breathe* and now *Feel*? What's with all this touchy-feely stuff? Do I need to hold you and stroke your back tenderly?

JS: I've been thinking about the importance of our readers understanding that paleo is not just a way or eating or moving, sleeping or playing. It's like we said in the first chapter, it is a Tao - a way of bringing you into harmony with yourself, and everything around you.

JG: Yes, you're right - the food you eat, the way you sleep, the way you play, the way you move, the way you feel, they are all just steps along the path to your Tao...but you didn't answer my questions.

JS: I think it's important to add in a short chapter about the concept of *Feel* and about what *The Tao of Paleo* really means. This subject might be a bit too serious for our usual modus operandi with fictitious characters, so we should probably tackle it alone. To answer your last question, touch me and I'll scream.

JG: Like a little girl, no doubt. OK, go ahead and elaborate on *Feel*.

JS: So part of the idea here is to develop a healthy relationship with your with food, but also with your body and your mind, and to understand that finding your Tao will require you to do more than "go on a diet." Many people are driven to try to find their paleo Tao strictly because they have an unhealthy connection with food and a poor body image. Maybe they can't eat at all without guilt, frustration, and some degree of self-loathing. Those people typically approach paleo thinking what most people think: That it is a diet to help them lose weight and that the quantity of food consumed is the sole factor in determining their body composition and their success.

JG: Quantity of food is one factor, undoubtedly, but it's not that simple. Finding your path to health and harmony is much more involved. Quality of food, gender, age, hormones, sleep, play, stress, exercise, and macronutrient proportions are all important players. There is no single formula for everyone.

JS: Yes. Finding your Tao isn't simply a matter of "eat this, do that" and you will magically morph into a supermodel.

JG: I hear that.

JS: Finding your Tao is going to require a paradigm shift from the failed concept of "going on a diet" to the authentic process of "changing your life." It takes longer than just a month or two to stop thinking about popcorn and baguettes, to replace the scale with an honest assessment of how you feel, and to abandon the programming that tells us that putting calories in our mouths makes us fat.

It takes a while to learn to trust our body's signals and instincts. It will require some time to learn feel confident about consuming significant amounts of food and eating when you are hungry.

One has to learn to abandon micromanaging the relationship with the scale on a daily basis.

JG: It takes some time - and as much headwork and heartwork as bodywork- to get into the groove with all this stuff. People have to "unlearn what they have learned," as Master Yoda would say, after years of thinking about food, exercise, sleep, stress, and play in deeply flawed ways.

JS: It's important to trust what you're doing as well. Physical changes don't always happen quickly, and we are all conditioned to expect the quick fix. We may have a day of less-than-perfect eating and look in the mirror the next day and think, in a state of panic, that what we are doing isn't working. The reality is that it is way too soon to conclude anything.

JG: We have found that there are a lot of people who can't give themselves permission to feel better, to look better, and be healthier. We understand that there are deep-seated emotional issues behind this, but the bottom line is that you should learn to accept certain facts.

JS: That's right. You have to believe that there is nothing inherently wrong with you or your body or your genes. You need to internalize that you have every right to be a fit, healthy, happy, and awesome specimen of humanity.

There's another side of the emotional coin, too - many people who have lived their whole lives embarrassed by the person in the mirror often suddenly find that they are more attractive and are getting a lot more attention from others, from potential suitors, friends, family, co-workers, and even from strangers. It can be confusing, difficult, overwhelming. We are talking about overhauling your self-image, not just your body. You could possibly cure a lifelong disease that you have struggled really hard to learn to live with.

JG: It's not always an easy transition for people to make. I have experienced and understand that myself. Psychologically, it tends to be worse for women than for us guys because of the societal pressures placed on women to look a certain way. When change happens, it can be a significant shock.

JS: Good call. There's nothing wrong with getting a little professional assistance if you need it. Joe and I know several excellent people who specialize in helping their clients overcome emotional hurdles on the way to finding their Tao. We'll talk about them more specifically in the Resources chapter.

JG: Ok Joe, you've convinced me. I see why we need a chapter on *Feel*. Let's get going!

JS: Jason, we just finished.

JG: We did?

JS: Yep, we let everyone know that the first step on the path to finding your Tao is getting your mind right.

JG: By adjusting how you perceive yourself, right? By internalizing your own value and your absolute right to take control of your health and happiness.

JS: Yep. You got it. And by gradually learning to trust your instincts and appetite.

JG: Once you get rolling, you will build a new person the paleo way - from the inside out.

JS: You won't just "lose weight on a diet." You will start to put yourself in harmony with yourself and the Universe.

JG: This is deep bro. We need a clever way to end the chapter though.

JS: I have to get on a Skype call, really, so that will have to do.

JG: Really? After all that deep, significant sharing, you're just going to go off and Skype someone, just like that? No cuddling?

JS: Nope.

JG: You really hurt my feelings, you know that? Can I touch your cheek gently, with just a finger?

JS: You're about to get slapped.

CHAPTER FOURTEEN: THE PLAN

"Get a new plan, Stan." ~ Simon and Garfunkel, Fifty Ways to Leave Your Lover

"Everyone's got a plan until they get hit." ~ Joe Louis

JS: In the last 160 pages or so, we've thrown a lot of information your way. We've talked food, exercise, play, and rest. We've touched on carbs, fats, proteins, and supplements. We've given you a friendly reminder not to get too absorbed in the dogma and not to to sweat the small stuff, and we've talked about the mental aspect of change.

JG: Along the way, we've also trotted out a few silly figments of our imagination to help illustrate our points, teased each other mercilessly, and probably offended every major category of human, big or small, to one extent or another.

JS: It's been unbelievably fun.

JG: It really has. Since the first few pages, we've tried to make it clear that while there are certain overriding principles, each of you is ultimately going to have to discover your own unique path. You're going to have to find your Tao.

JS: Right. So in this chapter, what we are going to do is stop theorizing and explaining and present you with an actual template.

JG: We've used this plan extensively with our friends and family. We believe that following it will help you get healthy and lead you to find your own Tao.

JS: Eventually, you'll discover what is unique about your own Tao of Paleo. You might eat certain foods that some of us don't. You might have a different exercise plan that works best for you. You will develop your own unique style of play.

JG: Look at this template like a signpost pointing to the start of your own paleo path. Like a finger pointing at the moon.

JS: All that being said, like we've repeated a few times, we respectfully suggest that you do your best to follow this template closely for a while. At the very least, it should get you metabolically healthy and flexible. It should boost your energy, it should get you established in a sustainable, effective fitness program, and it should leave you feeling great.

JG: The very first piece of preparation you need to do doesn't involve eating, sleeping, exercise, or playing.

JS: The very first work you need to do will occur between your ears and in your heart. As we discussed in *Feel,* many people have complex spiritual and mental issues with issues of food, fitness, and overall health.

JG: For many of us these issues are serious and real, and that they require inner strength and sometimes outside help to overcome.

JS: Unless you are mentally prepared to accept the fact that you can and have every right to be healthy, fit, and well, and to look it on the outside, it's going to be very difficult for you to benefit from this template, and even more difficult for you to eventually find your own Tao.

JG: If you feel that you need an ace in the hole in terms of mental and spiritual coaching, our friend Cinnamon Prime (yes that really is her real name, not just her superhero name), nutritionist, coach, and overall mind ninja, might be the perfect solution. You could also check out another old friend, Jackie Chatman, who heads up Eating for Wellness, a health retreat and counseling program in Southern California. Jackie is highly skilled at helping her clients learn proper nutrition and exercise, and she's a superstar when it comes to helping others deal with emotional and stress issues related to food, self-image, and habit patterns. We've included the contact information for both of them in the *Resources* chapter of the book.

JS: Cinnamon and Jackie pretty much rock.

JG: Damn straight.

JS: Onward and upward.

JG: Once you are mentally prepared for a health transformation, the next item on your checklist is to prepare yourself for thirty days of strict paleo eating. The purpose of this step is to teach your body to stop being dependent on easily accessible sources of glucose and to relearn how to burn fat for energy. Any cheating, consumption of sweetened paleo "treats" or even consumption of excess amounts of fruit could derail or delay this process, so once you start, go hardcore and stay the course.

JS: The thirty-day period will also begin the process of healing your gut and digestive system, which needs to recover from years of damage from the Standard American Diet.

GG: (Moaning) Graiiiins! BRAIIINS!

JG: Didn't you cut him in half with a chain saw a few chapters ago?

JS: Those zombies are pretty tough. Here, try this twelve-gauge.

JG: (cocking and locking) Hasta La Vista Grainiak!

KABOOM!!

JS: I'd say that did the trick.

JG: Ewwww! Zombie guts and partially digested grains everywhere.

JS: We'll clean up later. Back to the plan.

JG: Right. If you live on your own, we recommend you go through your closets and refrigerator and kick all those non-paleo foods to the curb. This will eliminate temptation and make your thirty-day kickstart easier. Donate nonperishables to a charity organization. With the caveat that they shouldn't eat any of it. Ever.

JS: If you have a spouse, partner and/or other family living with you, ask them if they will be willing to try the first thirty days along with you. If your significant others aren't ready to give the paleo lifestyle a try and you have to go it on your own, sit down with them and let them know how important it is for you to get healthy. Tell them that you need their help and support. This might mean a significant amount of inconvenience for them as you will be eating separate meals at the very least, so be sensitive to their role in your journey. Hopefully, they will reconsider when they witness your transformation.

JG: Right you are. OK. After you've set the date to start your thirty days of strict paleo, put together a shopping list. As a reminder, here's a helpful summary of Yes, No, and In Moderation foods:

YES:
- Animal protein (preferably organic, grass-fed, and or pastured), including but not limited to: Beef, pork, lamb, chicken, turkey, wild-caught fish, and shellfish. Fatty cuts are encouraged and preferred. Processed meats like sausage and bacon are excellent as well as long as they are chemical, sugar, and gluten-free. Organ meats are particularly nutrient-dense and easy on the budget.
- Eggs (avoid soy/vegetarian fed, look for pastured, if not, then cage free and/or organic).
- Green vegetables (organic).
- Starchy vegetables (sweet potatoes, squashes, parsnips, turnips, taro root, Brussels sprouts).
- Mushrooms.
- Fruit (particularly berries, cantaloupe, and other relatively low-fructose fruits).
- Fermented products (sauerkraut, kombucha).
- Spices and some condiments, including hot sauces, Worcestershire (check ingredients first), mustards, vinegars, and coconut aminos.
- Guacamole (check to make sure ingredients are clean).
- Organic extra virgin coconut oil (for cooking).
- Ghee/clarified butter or regular butter (for cooking).
- Extra virgin olive oil (for raw use only).
- Avocado oil (for cooking).
- Coconut water.
- Paleo jerkies (we recommend Steve's Original Paleo Products, Nick's Sticks, and Epic Bars).
- Quality canned seafood (we like Wild Planet products).

- Sea salt (ideally Himalayan, but anything that that has no additives - add lots in the first few weeks to offset all the sodium you were getting from baked goods).

NO:
- Grains and cereals of any kind, including wheat, barley, rye, rice, quinoa, or corn. White rice can be added later, if tolerated, for active people.
- Pastas.
- Legumes, including beans and peanuts.
- Seed and vegetable oils, such as canola, grapeseed, corn, or flaxseed.
- Soy, or any product that contains it.
- White potatoes. They can be added later (without skins) if tolerated.
- Dairy products, including cheese, milk or yogurt.
- Sugar, or sugar equivalents and substitutes (saccharin, corn syrup, aspartame, Splenda, stevia, agave nectar). Honey, maple syrup, or molasses can be added back in, in moderation, later.
- Processed foods that have chemical ingredients you don't recognize.
- Chips, crisps, candies, or "snack" foods.
- Sodas of any kind.
- Fruit juices
- Beer, whiskeys, wine, or distilled spirits

IN MODERATION:
- Raw nuts (almonds, walnuts, macadamias, pecans, pistachios).
- Nut butters (almond, cashew).
- High fructose fruits (bananas, apples, pears).
- Heavy cream.
- Coffee.
- 85% cacao or higher dark chocolate (as few additives as possible).
- High level predator fishes such as tuna and swordfish (due to contamination).
- Nightshades (peppers, tomatoes, tomatillos, eggplants).

JG: If you are suffering from an autoimmune disease, we strongly recommend that you avoid nightshades, nuts, and fructose altogether. They can aggravate your symptoms.

JS: If you stick with the recommendations above, you'll be on solid paleo ground. However, you might be one of those people like Jason that actually reads the directions when you assemble IKEA furniture and you need a bit more detailed guidance.

JG: You might be a creative, food-porn watching, cheffy type and feel very comfortable going into your kitchen with the list above, turning on the stove, brandishing some pricey cutlery, shouting "BAM!" a few times, and creating sumptuous paleo meals. On the other hand, you might be a bit more culinarily-challenged. You might want some recipes. You may even like the idea of a complete meal plan for your thirty-day kickoff and beyond.

JS: We've included a three month meal plan with loads of delicious paleo recipes from our dear friend Orleatha Smith in the Appendix. We encourage you to try them. Orleatha holds a master's in education and is a holistic nutritionist and a wonderful chef who honed her culinary skills cooking for her family.

JG: Thanks Orleatha! (Joe and Jason do The Wave back and forth in their chairs four times)

JS: We also love Sara Fragoso, paleo chef extraordinaire. Her *Everyday Paleo* series of paleo-friendly cookbooks is a great resource. It's well worth the price to pick up a couple of her books.

JG: If you're going to put together meals on your own, be as creative as you like. Just remember that your plate should contain mostly animal protein, green leafy vegetables, and fats, with modest servings of approved starchy vegetables, and low-fructose fruits.

JS: Let's talk about what your experience might be like when you actually start. It may well be that your thirty-day transition to the paleo lifestyle is easy from a dietary point of view, but if you're like most people, including me, the first few days can be challenging.

JG: You struggled with the carb flu didn't you, Joe?

JS: Yep. My body was addicted to grains and sugary carbs that it could easily convert to glucose. For those first few days my body was begging for sugar. I was foggy and less energetic than usual. It felt like someone had sucked my brains out my nose.

JG: Ewww. Like the way they made the mummies in Ancient Egypt.

JS: Exactly. I stuck with it though, making sure I ate plenty of good, quality paleo-friendly food, especially fats. Before I knew it the carb flu had passed and I felt amazing. My body was becoming fat-adapted I was and finally learning to access those fat stores for energy.

JG: This brings us to another important point. You have probably been told all your life that calorie restriction is the secret to weight loss and health. You've probably got your little food scale out, ready to weigh portions of food down to the quarter ounce.

JS: Put that sucker away. You won't be needing it.

JG: Practicing calorie restriction may cause you to lose weight, but it will also create hormonal and metabolic problems that will make it very difficult to maintain the weight loss when you restore normal calorie intake. It will likely also result in the loss of critical muscle mass, effectively robbing you of an important fat-burning tool.

Most people who go on calorie-restricted diets gain back some or all of the lost weight later on due to these two factors.

If you try to calorie restrict, you'll also probably feel like garbage, what with the low energy levels caused by your body's hormonal reaction to the stress. That's most un-paleo.

JS: So when you eat, don't count calories or limit your portions. As long as you are eating in accordance with the template, eat when you are hungry and until you are no longer hungry. Don't keep shoveling away because you like the taste.

JG: As time goes on you may find it beneficial to eat all your calories in one or two meals, during an eight hour window in the middle of the day. For many people, this is the optimum window from a fat-burning point of view. You'll figure that out later. For now, don't worry too much about it, as long as you aren't waking up ravenous in the middle of the night. In fact, ditch the scale completely. It will only thwart your ability to find your Tao.

JS: If you are waking up to eat, that could be sign that you're not eating enough or that you have a hormonal imbalance. If the former, you need to eat more good, quality paleo food at mealtimes. If the latter, you need to work on lowering stress, getting more sunlight during the day time, and cutting out blue light after sunset.

JG: We want to make sure you don't limit portions or count calories, but it's also critical that you don't skimp on fat. Good-quality saturated fat is absolutely essential to maintaining a healthy metabolism.

JS: It's also a natural mood elevator. Enjoy the fatty cuts of meat, eat your bacon, cook in generous helpings of coconut oil and ghee, and spoon out generous sides of (clean) guacamole.

JG: It's a myth that eating healthy saturated fats will make you fatter, or raise your cholesterol. Just the opposite, actually. It's the intake of processed foods, excessive sugar, and grains that make you retain fat.

JS: We also don't want you to eliminate carbohydrates. Remember, this isn't Atkins.

JG: Nope, not at all. Although it's true that if your goal is to burn a lot of fat, it makes sense to limit fruits and starchy vegetables like sweet potatoes, parsnips, turnips, and squash to sensible amounts, you still need to eat them. If you are active it's really important to eat even more carbs in order to restore glycogen levels, maintain hormonal balance, and prevent that nasty muscular catabolism.

JS: Very true.

CC: And THAT'S a'why you need to eat a BIG PLATE of my PASTA!!

JG: Did you untie her??

JS: Are you kidding me?? No way.

CC: I ate'a my way through the fettuccini, you gnocchi-hating knuckleheads! I'mma BACK, biyatches!

JS: Uh-oh!

JG: Better clench up Legolas.

JS: It's Joe, and what's with the grey robes, staff, and conical hat?

JG: (yelling) You cannot pasta!! I am a server of the secret steak, a wielder of the fork of Carnivore! You cannot pasta!! The egg noodles will not avail you! Flame of Udon! Go back to the shadows! YOU CANNOT PASTA!!

JS: Great. Not only is this going to go over about fifty percent of your heads, now we're looking at a lawsuit from the Tolkien family AND Peter Jackson.

CC: AHHHHH! I'm melllllting! What a world, what a world, what a world...

JS: And now L. Frank Baum's estate. Wow. Nothing left but a puddle of tomato sauce and a pile of semolina flour.

JG: Fly, you fools.

JS: Yeah, you've beat that one like a redheaded step-orc. Let's talk about our experiments with low carbohydrates.

JG: Sure. Both of us experimented with low-carb eating for a while - trying to keep our carbs in the 30-50 gram per day range. In my case, it was a disaster. I leaned out briefly, but then immediately saw my cortisol levels spike upward. My levels of leptin - a hormone produced in the hypothalamus that regulates the sensation of fullness and helps metabolize fat, dropped severely. Within a few weeks I had replaced some of that belly fat I had worked so hard to eliminate, I was sleeping poorly, I had bad muscle cramps, and my energy level dropped like a stone.

JS: I tried the same thing, and basically drove myself into a state of hormonal imbalance and fatigue. I couldn't exercise without getting exhausted. I couldn't recover properly from workouts. My muscles felt like Play-Doh.

JG: Did you use them to mold cool and interesting shapes like dinosaurs, or space aliens?

JS: No, I did not. But I began to recover when I restored sensible amounts of carbohydrates from fruits and starchy vegetables to my diet.

JG: Me too. After a few weeks of normal carb intake I was back in business.

JS: I'm never going low-carb again.

JG: Me neither. I'd rather slow dance with a warthog.

JS: Warthog slow dancing is no one's idea of The Tao of Paleo.

JG: True dat. That being said, as we mentioned in *Carbs,* if you are diabetic, sedentary, or if you have significant amounts of excess body fat to burn, you may be one of the minority that benefit from a low-carb diet. We'd like to emphasize that in our experience, that's the exception rather than the rule, and as you lean out, it makes less and less metabolic sense to maintain a low-carb regime.

JS: Let's talk about the exercise template. By the time you're a few weeks into your thirty day kickstart, you're probably going to have energy to burn. We recommend that until you start to feel that energy, you restrict yourself to the long, slow, walks we talked about in *Move* to avoid stressing your body as it makes the transition to becoming fat-adapted.

Keep in mind that the walking is highly effective metabolically, you should plan on taking these types of walks over the long term, hopefully till you hit one hundred and ten. Walking should be thought of as an addition to your formal exercise plan.

JG: Walk at first. Once you feel energetic, however, there's no reason why you can't begin a program of paleo-centric exercise.

CC: Yes! It's time to start Cardio! Give me a "C!" Give me an "A!" Give me a "RDIO!"

JG: It's Claudio again. Yay.

JS: What's a freaking RDIO? Hold on, I'll fix this.

JG: Nice Joe! You pantsed him!!

CC: GAARGGGH! I am so embarrassed!

JS: I would be too if I were wearing a EuroDisney Mickey Mouse man thong.

JG: Look at him trying to run away with his pants around his ankles.

JS: Bye Claudio. Run along now.

JG: I think we've seen the last of him.

JS: As we were saying before we were so rudely interrupted, we'd suggest that you try a two to three-day per week program when you're starting to feel frisky. One workout should be a series of short sprints followed by brief periods of recovery. If you're not up to running, you can do these sprints on an ergometer - a rowing machine - or even on an elliptical runner or stair machine.

JG: The key is short duration and intervals of 80%+ effort and rest. Perhaps you can start with ten to twenty second sprints alternating with twenty-second walks. Try this for eight cycles and make sure you warm up and cool down. You can knock this workout out in ten minutes.

JS: If you can't complete eight at first, that's fine. As time goes on, you can lengthen the duration of the sprints and the number of cycles, but don't go nuts. Short duration is key for fat burning and to ensure you don't run out of glycogen.

JG: For your second workout, we'd recommend a session of lifting heavy weights, focusing on the big lifts like squats, cleans, deadlifts, and/or presses. Again we recommend that

after your warmup, you exert at least 80% effort in each set. Because these full-body lifts are demanding and technique can break down quickly as you tire, it's a good idea to go for low-repetition sets, either in a pyramid sequence (5 reps, 3 reps, 1 rep, 3 reps, then 5 reps again), or as you become more advanced, single lifts near maximum effort.

JS: As we mentioned before, the first step is to make sure your form is solid. If you aren't familiar with these lifts and aren't proficient in performing them safely, you need to invest in some time with a good trainer who can get you in the groove.

JG: If you aren't comfortable with any trainers in your geographical area, we have a few suggestions. We've mentioned our friend Cinnamon Prime, who is based in the Dallas/Fort Worth, Texas area. Cinnamon can help you with your exercise regimen regardless of your physical location. Darryl Edwards, whom we introduced you to in *Play*, is a skilled paleo-centric trainer based in the UK but travels widely and trains clients all over the world. You could also consider taking advantage of Jason Seib and Sara Fragoso's EPLifefit program. Their excellent professionals can train you online using innovative and effective technology. We've included the contact information for these terrific experts in our *Resources* section.

JS: We talked earlier about the importance of mobility and joint flexibility. We'd like to recommend that you begin a flexibility program concurrent with your weight workouts. In *Move* we mentioned Dr. Kelly Starrett, author of *Becoming a Supple Leopard.* We encourage you to buy this book. At the very least, check out Dr. Starett's website at www.mobilitywod.com for some simple mobility routines.

JG: The kind of joint flexibility and set of solid braced positions that you can acquire from a good mobility program are indispensable to exercising safely.

JS: To put it very simply, if you go hard without maintaining the necessary flexibility and good body position, you're not going to get all the benefit from your workouts and you may get hurt.

JG: We don't recommend getting hurt. If you are a masochist, you're in the wrong book. Go in the back section and look for the spiked books with the leather hoods.

JS: There's a back section??? Where???

JG: You're not old enough to go in the back.

JS: Lame. Oh well.

JG: If you're interested in some serious fat burning, you can add a short High Intensity Interval Training (HIIT) workout once per week. Pick a set of exercises that preferably involve full-body movements. I like to use pushups, pull-ups, crunches, box jumps, short ergometer sprints, burpees, kettlebell swings, or similar options.

As an example of a HIIT session, you might pick six of these exercises. After a thorough warmup, proceed to do complete circuits of the movements you have chosen, with little or no rest in between, until time has expired. Finish with a thorough cool down.

JS: Although HIIT sessions are awesome fat burners, they are absolutely not recommended for people who are significantly overweight or at lower levels of fitness. Even advanced paleo HIIT ninjas like Jason never exceed twenty minutes in their HIIT sessions. We recommend that you start with a session of eight to ten minutes unless you are already very fit and used to this type of training.

JG: Right. In fact, as we mentioned before, if you have substantial amounts of fat to lose, if you have significant improvements to make in the area of flexibility, or you're not used to exercise, it's perfectly reasonable that you hold off on all of these types of sessions and limit your workouts to slow walking until you've gotten healthier. Perhaps then you might like to hire a trainer to slowly introduce you to the types of workouts we've described. Everyone has to find the Tao that suits them best. Even without strenuous exercise, this template should yield impressive results.

JS: Tying the workouts and nutrition together. If you ARE going to work out rigorously, especially if you are going to do HIIT, we can't stress enough that you need to maintain an appropriate carb intake to fuel your activity. Try to eat some starchy carbs like sweet potatoes at each meal in order to replenish glycogen levels and prevent muscle catabolism and bonking - hitting a wall and running out of energy during exercise.

JG: Bonking is no fun. I'd rather snuggle with a Gila monster.

JS: Gila monster snuggling is not recommended.

JG: One more thing. Let's say one day you had a poor night of sleep, or you're under the weather. The traditional exercise ethos says that if you aren't feeling tippy-top, you should suck it up and head to the gym anyway, you wimp, after all, do you want to miss a workout and spontaneously gain fifty pounds of ugly fat overnight and completely destroy your value as a human being, you filthy, disgusting…

JS: Jason…

JG: Sorry. I get carried away.

JS: You think???

JG: The point is, this thinking is completely flawed from a scientific point of view. If you've had a poor night of sleep or you're not feeling well, your body is already under a higher than normal amount of unwanted stress.

JS: We've beat you over the head with the hormonal and metabolic outcomes of excessive stress. If you've missed it so far, here's the Cliff's Note: Excessive stress is going to result in a whole bunch of non-fun, un-paleo effects on your body, mind, and spirit, which causes more stress and can spiral all the way to disease if it gets far enough.

JG: Yep. If you're feeling less than good, don't make a bad situation worse by stressing your body further with strenuous exercise. Take a walk instead and focus on eating well, relaxing, and getting a good night's sleep.

JS: Tomorrow's another day. Don't lose sight of the big picture. The idea of this whole paleo path is to make your life better, healthier, and more satisfying. Beating yourself to a pulp in the gym when you're sick and tired isn't very paleo.

JG: I think we pretty much beat exercise and movement to a pulp. Shall we press on and talk about play?

JS: Whatever you say playa.

JG: Spend time prior to your paleo start date doing some serious reflection on how you want to play, because we're going to ask that you add regular play sessions to your thirty-day kickoff.

Play is important in a biochemical sense because it alleviates stress, of course. But pulling back again and looking at the big picture, the goal is to lead a happier and more enjoyable life. What's more wonderful than giving yourself a chance to play??

TT: Don't listen to these fools!! You can't waste your time playing!! You'll miss out on everything important at WORK! WORK!! WORK!!!!

JS: All these people are going to show up again, aren't they?

JG: It appears so.

JS: Shall we handle it as usual?

JG: Still got your fiddle?

JS: Right here next to my liter of duck fat.

JG: And a one, and a two, and a three: "Spin your partner round again, clap your hands and count to ten! Eat some chicken, roast some duck, now take your partner and go…"

JS: Woah!!! What about our G rating????

JG: I was going to say "go drive a truck."

JS: Ah, I see.

JG: Looks like Terrence is square-dancing off over the horizon.

JS: Let's hope we taught him something.

JG: Wouldn't bet a fiddle of gold against your soul on it.

JS: Mega-unfunny.

JG: Back to play?

JS: Yes, please.

JG: It sounds lame, but what we'd like you to do is sit down and make a list of things you really enjoy doing. They can be mental or physical or a combination of both, and it's okay if your line between exercise and play is a bit blurry.

JS: Just like Jason.

JG: If you can't immediately identify things that make you happy, try to make it basic and simple. Maybe you enjoy taking your dog out for a stroll, or playing with your kids in the park, or sitting and listening to classical music.

Take the opportunity to list some things that you don't do, but have always wanted to try. Maybe you're interested in learning to sail, or play croquet, or do needlepoint, or play the xylophone. Make arrangements to try some of these things.

JS: We'd like you to set aside at least three hours per week for scheduled play during your thirty-day kickoff. If you're able to do some spontaneous play on top of that, all the better. Maybe you end up running under the sprinkler with your kids or throwing a frisbee around with your roommates on the spur of the moment, or you indulge in an impromptu snowball fight. Look for these opportunities as they present themselves and take advantage of them!

JG: Make sure that however you choose to play, pick activities that take you away from the stress of everyday life and allow you a period of mental vacation. You'll be amazed at how this helps both your progress toward your physical goals and your overall happiness.

We'd like to remind you again about our friend Darryl Edwards, trainer, nutritionist, and all-around awesome bloke from Merry Olde England. He's an expert in the restorative power of play, and he is also the founder of a system called PRIMALity, which uses play to create healthier, fitter humans. Darryl travels all over the world doing seminars and presentations, and he might be able to help you to reconnect with your inner paleoplayful self. His contact information is in the *Resources* section.

JS: Ok I think we pimped out Darryl enough.

JG: At least for a few more pages. We just dig his approach.

JS: And we've talked about setting the table for your thirty-day kickoff by getting your mind right and your pantry nice and paleo-ready. We've discussed what to eat and what to avoid. We've covered exercise. We've touched on the importance of play. There's one more important thing we need to mention.

JG: The Lambada?

JS: No.

JG: It's the Forbidden Dance, you know.

JS: Yes, I'm aware. But we're going to talk about sleep.

JG: Oh. Not the Lambada.

JS: You're going to read what we tell you next and you might say "I was with you guys up to this point but you just lost me."

JG: Yep. You're gonna be all "THAT ain't gonna happen."

JS: What we are going to tell you is we'd like you to get at least eight hours of sleep per night in a pitch-dark room. Not just for your thirty-day kickoff, but for the rest of your life.

JG: Now there will be a brief intermission while we allow you to laugh until your ribs hurt and then wipe the tears from your eyes.

JS: Hmmmm, hmmmm, hmmmm, hmm-h-hmmm, hmm-h-hmmm...

JG: What are you humming?

JS: Intermission music.

JG: That's the Darth Vader theme from Star Wars.

JS: I really like the Darth Vader theme from Star Wars.

JG: I think they've finished laughing and wiping their eyes now, so let's continue. Listen: Joe and I get it. You have a stressful job. You need to unwind when you get home. There's family to spend time with. There might be a second job or a ton of housework. You might think eight hours of sleep is just a pipe dream.

JS: It's really important, though. Starting with the obvious: if you get sufficient sleep, you're going to feel better, have more energy, and generally feel healthier and happier than if you don't get sufficient sleep.

JG: Right…which is all very paleo.

WW: This is absolute malarky. I drink seven double cafe frappa-dappa-chino espressos after nine o'clock at night every night, slay zombies on my custom gaming console, check my email, work out, sleep two or three hours, wake up, walk around with a latte IV in my arm, and I feel amazing.

JS: Here we go again.

WW: Sleep is overrated. I'll get plenty of sleep when I'm dead.

JG: Which is probably going to be very soon the way you're going.

JS: Hey Wilma Wired, look what I've got for you! It's a new cup of hybrid coffee, with seven times the normal amount of caffeine. I call it the Espressageddon.

WW: OOOOHH! GIMME GIMME!

JS: Here you go.

WW: Gluggluggglugglug! WHOA I am SOOOOO tired ZZZZZZZZZZ!

JG: Nicely done. What did you spike that with?

JS: My own special formula. She'll be out for a while.

JG: Back to sleep, then. Or rather, let's wake up to the importance of those eight hours from a metabolic point of view. The scientific evidence is mounting that eight hours or more of uninterrupted sleep has a massive impact on hormonal levels.

JS: As we discussed in *Sleep* you need to avoid electronics around bedtime to make sure you're not getting too much blue light, and you need to stay away from alcohol, strenuous exercise, and large meals close to bedtime.

JG: Yep.

JS: We've knocked you over the head about cortisol enough times for you to understand that elevated cortisol levels can lead to your body hoarding fat and burning muscle instead.

JG: As an example, a 1997 study published in *The Journal of Sleep Research and Sleep Medicine* focusing on sleep and cortisol levels was pretty conclusive and typical in its findings. A test group of healthy young men was subjected to three separate sleep schedules - sleep deprivation, sleep interruption after four hours, and a normal eight hours of sleep. The sleep deprived group had cortisol levels 45% higher than the normal sleep group twenty-four hours after the period of deprivation, while the interrupted sleep group had levels 37% higher than the normal sleep group.

JS: Back to the two other hormones that are critical to the metabolic process: leptin and ghrelin. To dramatically oversimplify, leptin signals the body that it is satiated and doesn't need any more to eat, while ghrelin stimulates the appetite, especially for sugary carbohydrates.

JG: Failing on those eight hours plays havoc with your leptin and ghrelin levels. It's going to make it so much harder to eat what your body actually needs and make it far harder to make good food choices.

Again, the science is convincing. A 2004 Stanford University/ University of Wisconsin study which sampled over one thousand subjects found that there was a direct relationship between getting less than eight hours of sleep and having elevated ghrelin and low leptin levels. Participants who got five hours of sleep had leptin levels 15.5% lower than those who got eight hours, and the five hour sleepers had ghrelin levels 14.8% higher. More significantly, participants who reported averaging five hours of sleep had BMI (Body Mass Indexes) 3.6% higher than those who got eight hours of sleep (when adjusted for age, weight, and sex) showing a correlation between these altered hormone levels, lack of sleep, and weight gain.

JS: It's about more than feeling better. We went all sciencey on you there for a while to show you that those eight hours of sleep are tremendously important in terms of succeeding with this template and finding your Tao.

JG: Using electronics shortly before bedtime can also interrupt restful sleep. So try to turn off the TV, the computer, and all your toys well before you hit the hay and get those eight hours of sleep. We think this is just as important as all the other parts of the template.

JS: Absolutely. Lack of adequate sleep could very well prevent you from reaching your goals and finding your Tao. Make it a priority. You will thank us later.

JG: We've just about covered it all, haven't we?

JS: Let's see, feelings, food, exercise, play and sleep. It sounds to me like we've touched all the bases. Except…

JG: I know exactly what you're thinking. Don't you dare.

JS: But you're breaking her heart.

JG: DO NOT bring that psycho poobah back in here.

JS: You're shaking her confidence daily.

JG: I mean it, Joe. No Cecilia. I'm as serious as a heart attack.

JS: Don't worry. I sent her to Vanuatu on a singles cruise. No making love in the afternoon for you with Cecilia up in your bedroom.

JG: I am gonna hurl.

JS: We've gone over the ins and outs of supplementation, but it's not a required part of the template. It may be a part of your individual Tao though, so we'll leave the decision on supplements to you. However, Jason and I both agree that you should get out in the sunlight and make sure you don't cheat your body of necessary vitamin D. If you're lucky enough to live in a warm part of the world, strip down to a bathing suit…

JG: Or less, if you're Joe.

JS: …and spend some time outside.

JG: I think now, we're really, really done.

JS: Looks that way.

JG: How do we end this thing?

JS: I think, pretty much just like we started.

JG: Hey Joe! Look at that night sky. And check out that moon! Isn't it gorgeous???

JS: Where?

JG: Over there dude! Look at where I'm pointing! See, with my finger!

JS: All I can see is your finger.

JG: Sigh.

CHAPTER FIFTEEN: RESOURCES

"What has it got in its nasty little pocketses?" ~ Gollum

JS: What, indeed, precious?

JG: Creepy.

JS: Yep. So now we're at the part of the book where we want to put some pretty cool stuff in your paleo pocketses.

JG: Nicely turned.

JS: Thank you. Basically, what we're going to do is give you some tools that will help you along as you set off in search of your paleo Tao.

JG: To help you on your unexpected journey.

JS: You're making a hobbit of aggravating the Tolkien estate. And I hear they are very litigious.

JG: That's a bad bad hobbit…OK, OK. No more of those references.

JS: We're going to start with a series of WEBSITES and BOOKS that we believe are of excellent general interest and will help the paleo newbie and the grizzled grass-fed guzzler alike. And no one paid us to put these in here - they are here because they are good solid, trusted sources and can really help you.

JG: The alliteration store called and they want it all back.

JS: Tough titty. First and foremost we'd like to direct you to *The Tao of Paleo* website at www.paleotao.com. Jason and I will continue to shock, awe, and amaze you with a stunning series of superb articles, blog posts, and podcasts.

JG: You're not going to stop, are you?

JS: You can have my alliterations when you pry them from my frozen, grass-fed fingers.

JG: Next, we'd like to recommend the website of one of the true titans of The Paleo Movement...

JS: It's contagious, isn't it?

JG: Robb Wolf. Robb, originally a research chemist, is an accomplished nutritionist, author of the bestseller *The Paleo Solution*, and the co-owner of NorCal Fitness. Robb's website at www.robbwolf.com is a terrific repository of knowledge on every aspect of the paleo lifestyle.

JS: Sitting up there with Robb in the Paleo Pantheon is Mark Sisson.

JG: Mark is a former elite long distance runner and triathlete. His *Primal Blueprint* series of books are a must read, although his primal take on nutrition is slightly different from orthodox paleo.

JS: Mark's blog, Mark's Daily Apple, at www.marksdailyapple.com, is an invaluable resource with a handy searchable database of Mark's concise and well-written articles and blog posts.

JG: **Dr. Loren Cordain is the granddaddy of the modern Paleo Movement. He essentially made the whole kit and caboodle famous with his bestselling book** *The Paleo Diet.* **The updated 2010 addition,** *The Paleo Answer,* **should most certainly be on your bookshelf, or in your electronic reader, or chiseled onto some stone tablets for you to carry around as you wander aimlessly through the desert.**

JS: Or whatever. It's a great book. Also visit Dr. Cordain's website at www.thepaleodiet.com

JG: **We've found two great websites that will allow you to connect with paleo friendly healthcare practitioners in your area. Primal Docs is a network of over eight hundred professionals around the country. You can find them at www.primaldocs.com**

JS: The Paleo Physician's Network, at www.paleophysiciansnetwork.com, is another key resource that will help you find health professionals who practice in a paleo way.

JG: **We'd also like to give a paleo shout out to Katy Haldiman, skilled nurse, podcaster, nutritional therapist, and personal trainer based in the Northern California Bay Area. Katy can help you make healing changes in your life through the power of real food. She consults worldwide via Skype. Find Katy at www.thepaleonurse.com or at www.paleocare.com**

JS: She's also brilliant, sexy, and an all-around totally awesome paleo babe.

JG: She happens to be Joe's significant other. Lucky dog, that Joe is.

JS: Woofity woof.

JG: If you're a Facebooker, we'd like to recommend you join The International Paleo Movement Group (IPMG). This online community is comprised of over twelve thousand members from around the world, ranging from the merely curious to the hardcore paleo nerd. Joe is one of the administrators of this group, and he'd be happy to welcome you aboard.

JS: Absolutely. There's no better place to meet new paleo friends and discuss any and every facet of the paleo lifestyle with your fellow tribe members. On a daily basis, group members post dozens of helpful links, interesting articles, inspiring progress photos, and tasty paleo recipes. You can find IPMG here: http://bit.ly/paleogroup

JG: If you're looking for inspiration, I might suggest a great book put together by a certain close friend of mine.

JS: You have one of those?

JG: I was talking about you, smarty pants.

JS: Oh. Well…considering the fact that you're about to give me a shameless plug, I'll allow the familiarity…this time.

JG: How generous of you. My friend Joe is the author of *The Paleo Miracle: 50 Real Stories of Health Transformation*. It's like paleo chicken soup for the soul.

JS: The book is a compilation of the stories of fifty-nine real people - each of whom saw their lives transformed after finding the paleo lifestyle. Many of them cured conditions like multiple sclerosis, heart disease, Hashimoto's, depression, ADHD, bipolar disorder, high blood pressure, and others, by finding their paleo

Tao. And I give a large portion of the profits to charity, just like Jason and I do with this book.

JG: Joe's story is in there too. And it has progress pictures!

JS: Mostly for people like you who don't read so good.

JG: What about people like you who don't grammar so good?

JS: Touché. Or threeché. What number are we on?

JG: Visit www.thepaleomiracle.com…and buy Joe's book. He really needs the money.

JS: Sigh.

JG: For a scientific yet accessible take on the paleo path, take a look at J. Stanton's www.gnolls.org. J is a talented paleo researcher and also an accomplished writer of fantasy novels. His website is filled with useful tidbits and thoughtful articles. And he is really tall.

JS: If you're the kind of paleo geek who enjoys reading research abstracts, we'd direct you to PubMed, a vast searchable database of articles and studies on biomedical research. You can get a first-hand look at all the studies we've mentioned in the book and dive deep into the science behind paleo. Visit Pubmed at www.ncbi.nlm.nih.gov/pubmed

JG: Finally we'd like to mention The Paleo Movement Online Magazine, at www.paleomovement.com. Our friend Karen Pendergrass, the Paleo Princess, has assembled an impressive website filled with interviews, tips, blog posts, recipes, and other useful stuff. It's updated weekly, and Joe sometimes posts there.

JS: I don't think she'd like being called a princess. More like a honey badger.

JG: Aren't there princess honey badgers?

JS: No.

JG: Fine. Visit the website anyway.

JS: Speaking of Pendergrasses, we also want to mention Karen's dad David Pendergrass, Ph.D. who teaches graduate biochemistry courses at Kansas University. He is an expert in the biochemistry of paleo. Dr. Pendergrass has a book coming out soon which he co-authored with Christina Lianos called *The Smartest Loser*. When it comes to understanding how food affects your brain, this book is fabulous. Check it out.

JG: And thanks to Dr. Pendergrass for scientific insight which helps move The Paleo Movement forward.

JS: Here here. OK, let's move on and talk about helping you find what to EAT. As we promised, we've got a complete three-month course of paleo recipes from our friend Orleatha Smith. You can find the meal plan in the back of this book.

JG: You can either follow the meal plan precisely or you can pick and choose recipes on an as-needed basis, or just save it for future reference if you're more of a do-it-yourself type.

JS: Exactly.

JG: Orleatha is a paleo holistic nutritionist par excellence. She's also an author, speaker, mom, and she holds a masters degree in education. Visit her website at www.lvlhealth.com

JS: We love us some Orleatha.

JG: We sure do.

JS: If you're looking for a great paleo cookbook, Jason and I love Sara Fragoso, pint-sized paleo powerhouse and master chef. Her *Everyday Paleo* series of cookbooks is filled with thousands of delicious recipes that are all solidly paleo. You can visit Sara's website at www.everydaypaleo.com

JG: When it comes to paleo vittles, our buddy Jadah Holland is another superstar. Her terrific blog, Salted Paleo, is filled with great recipes that Jadah either invents or kitchen-tests herself.

JS: Jadah's food pictures make my mouth water. As does Jadah herself.

JG: She's darned cute, that's for sure.

JS: Check out her website at www.relishscd.blogspot.com and tell her we sent you.

JG: At which point she will probably ban you.

JS: Nah. She likes us.

JG: Maybe.

JS: We'd be remiss if we didn't mention our good buddy Jimmy Moore.

JG: Especially since he wrote a foreword for the book.

JS: True.

JG: Jimmy is a bestselling author, podcaster, television personality, and blogger extraordinaire. His personal story is amazing - he lost over 180 pounds using the paleo template. His *Clarity* book series is a must read.

JS: He sure found his own Tao.

JG: Yep.

JS: Although many might benefit from a higher intake of carbs than Jimmy generally recommends, he's a legit luminary of The Paleo Movement. We highly recommend his books, including his most recent magnum opus *Cholesterol Clarity: What the HDL is wrong with my numbers?* This is the first book in his *Clarity* series and it's terrific. Visit Jimmy's website at www.livinlavidalowcarb.com

JG: Thanks again for the foreword, Jimmy. We left the money on the dresser.

JS: Hope you don't mind that it's in pennies.

JG: You might be asking yourself where to find all the high-quality meat, fish, poultry, fruit, and vegetables we mention ad infinitum.

JS: We suggest that you start by looking for local farmers. Often, grass-fed meat and organic fruits and veggies are closer than you think. Many farmers or groups of farmers have started meat-share programs, where you commit to weekly or monthly deliveries of seasonally available products for a fixed period of time. A good state-by-state directory can be found at www.eatwild.com

JG: Of course, you can visit your local grocery store. High quality chains like Wegman's, Whole Foods, and Trader Joe's have huge selections of well-raised meat and organic vegetables and fruit.

JS: Most supermarket chains are seeing the growing demand for quality food and have responded accordingly with larger organic food sections, and prices are steadily lowering.

JG: I travel for a living and that creates a number of paleo problems.

JS: Very true. We generally do not recommend you consume the preservative-laden food-like materials provided for your sustenance on airplanes, for example.

JG: Nope. If you travel, you're going to need a source of healthy paleo road chow. You might not be in a position to carry your own personal refrigerator around either, so it's likely that you'll need a source of nutrition that can be stored at room temperature.

JS: If you're fond of seafood, we recommend tinned wild-caught salmon, tuna, mackerel, or sardines from a reliable vendor like Wild Planet. Just open the can and add a little mustard, hot sauce, or the paleo-friendly condiment of your choice when it's time to mac out.

JG: If you prefer land-based vittles, consider buying a dehydrator and making your own grass-fed jerky or pemmican. It's not difficult. However if you consider that an overly ambitious project, Joe and I know of a few excellent purveyors of portable meat-meals.

JS: Steve's Original Paleo Goods is a favorite. They offer grass-fed beef and chicken jerkies and sticks as well as grainless crunch bars that are an excellent source of carbs. They will ship your order right to your home and it's always high quality. Check out their website at www.stevesoriginal.com

JG: A bag of jerky, some beef sticks, a crunch bar, and a few tablespoons of almond butter makes a solid paleo meal and saves you from the choice of either starving or ingesting something that only remotely resembles real food.

JS: One thing we love about Steve's is that they donate a large chunk of their revenues to Steve's Club - a fitness program for economically challenged, at-risk kids.

JG: Yep. A company with a mission and a heart.

JS: We can also recommend Epic bars - meat bars that come in your choice of beef, turkey, or bison. All three flavors are grass-fed/pastured, organic, and taste delicious.

JG: Epic will also ship their products to your door. Visit them at www.epic.com

JS: We also like Nick's Sticks, grass-fed beef and pastured turkey sticks from Nick Wallace of Wallace Farms, in Keystone, Iowa. Nick's Sticks are GMO, MSG, gluten, antibiotic and hormone-free. They are shelf-stable, reasonably priced, and they taste delicious. Order them online at www.nicks-sticks.com

JG: When it comes to learning how to MOVE, we've included a set of paleo workout templates at the end of the book. They are general in nature but they will give you a solid framework for your movement program. If you are unfamiliar with any of the exercises we mention, please contact a physical trainer you trust to demonstrate the proper techniques.

JS: That's a really important point. If you are inexperienced in exercise, or even unfamiliar with the workouts we're recommending, you absolutely need to hire a fitness professional to help you.

JG: Don't just walk into a gym and hire the first trainer you meet. Conduct your search like you would conduct a job interview. Get referrals from trusted sources. Make it clear that you want guidance in a paleo-centric exercise program - sprinting, lifting heavy weights, and moderate HIIT training.

JS: Make sure any trainer you consider is on board with these types of workouts, understands the basic paleo movement template, and is willing to train you in this way. If you start hearing about cardio, hour-long metcons, or spinning, you might want to politely walk away.

JG: Maybe back away slowly. They can smell your fear.

JS: If you are unable to find a local fitness professional that meets this criteria, we will recommend some excellent virtual options shortly. First, however, let's touch on something else.

JS: We mentioned how important it is to combine movement with flexibility. Before you initiate a workout program or look for a trainer, we'd highly recommend you invest in a copy of Dr. Kelly Starrett's *Becoming a Supple Leopard*.

JG: Kelly Starrett is a genius in the science of increasing human flexibility in order to optimize health and performance. You can learn more about Dr. Starrett and his revolutionary flexibility program on his website, www.mobilitywod.com.

JG: It's absolutely critical that you combine flexibility with movement in order to prevent injury and get the most out of your workouts.

JS: Yep. We can't go any further without reminding you about our friend Darryl Edwards, the Fitness Explorer, and his PRIMALity program.

JG: Darryl is not only a paleo nutritionist and author but also an expert in the area of physical training. His emphasis is on movements that improve your ability to perform daily, recreational, and extraordinary physical tasks effectively.

JS: He's passionate about helping humans recover their inborn sense of play, and reincorporating it into challenging and fun workouts. We love his book *Paleo Fitness*. You can check it out at www.amazon.com

JG: Darryl is based in London, UK, but he travels around the world conducting Primal Playouts and he can train you remotely regardless of your location.

JS: Not to mention he also wrote us a nice foreword for the book.

JG: And I didn't even have to dress up in my Britney Spears outfit and beg him.

JS: Fortunately for him. Check out Darryl's website at www.thefitnessexplorer.com or his Facebook page at www.facebook.com/fitnessexplorer

JG: We mentioned Sara Fragoso and her awesome *Everyday Paleo* recipe books, but along with her partner, Jason Seib, she also runs a virtual physical training program at www.eplifefit.com

JS: Jason is the owner of CPC Fitness and Fat Loss in Clackamas, Oregon and the author of *The Paleo Coach*, a stellar introduction to the paleo lifestyle.

JG: We love Jason and Sara's informative and entertaining free weekly podcast. And for reasonable rates, their staff of virtual trainers will provide you with all the expertise and personal attention you need to learn to work out effectively and safely.

JS: Sara, Jason, and EP Lifefit are the perfect choice for experienced paleo online training.

JG: When it comes to SLEEP we remind you how important quality rest is to becoming a healthy human.

JS: We think adequate sleep is perhaps the most underestimated aspect of finding your Tao. Remember that sleep has a tremendous effect on hormones like cortisol, leptin, ghrelin, and glucagon, which in turn, have a dramatic impact on your body composition and overall health. It's critical to get good, solid sleep.

JG: That's why we need to mention our friend Dan Koifman. He's a skilled sleep coach. He will teach you to master the mysteries of circadian rhythms and learn how to effectively biohack your body, all with the goal of helping you sleep better and more soundly.

JS: Dan's also an accomplished inventor, presently working on a set of glasses designed to enhance and improve rest. He's based in New York City but he consults virtually to clients located around the world.

JG: You can contact Dan at his Facebook page: www.facebook.com/dankoifman2

JS: You can't find your paleo Tao without mastering the mental game. Some of us need professional assistance to deal with the way we FEEL.

JG: You'll benefit from getting your mind right, just as you will from getting your diet, exercise, and sleep straightened out.

JS: Our friend Cinnamon Prime is a professional mindset coach.

JG: We also have our suspicions that she's actually a ninja. Or Batman. Or both.

JS: Coach Prime helps her clients rewire their brains so that they can better achieve their health and fitness goals.

JG: She's a master at helping you understand why you might have failed in the past and how to acquire the mindset to succeed in the future. She will teach you the ins and outs of paleo and exercise, empower you to create your own meal plans, and help you build a workout regimen.

JS: "This is not the food you're looking for."

JG: "This is not the food we're looking for."

JS: "Move along."

JG: **Your Jedi mind tricks won't work on me, boy. But Coach Prime's will work on everyone.**

JS: Most importantly, Coach's clients don't go on diets or exercise programs. They learn how to make permanent and lasting lifestyle changes.

JG: **You might even say that Coach illuminates the path to finding your paleo Tao.**

JS: She's like a bigass floodlight of righteous paleo candlepower.

JG: **Right on. Find Coach at her website - www.atruetransformation.com - or email her at info@atruetransformation.com. She is based in the Dallas/Fort Worth, Texas area, but she can work with you anywhere via phone, email, or Skype chat.**

JS: Or just look for her in the Bat Cave. Or wherever ninjas hang out when they aren't throwing sharp starry things at people.

JG: **We'd like to mention our buddy Jackie Chatman as well.**

JS: Aside from being a warm, wonderful lady, Jackie holds a masters degree in Clinical Psychology and a degree in holistic nutrition as well.

JG: **Jackie runs Eating for Wellness, a lovely retreat nestled in the warm desert springs of Southern California. She offers a four-day, three-night program that includes a comprehensive introduction to healthy eating with an eye toward a kindly and holistic approach to mental and physical health.**

JS: She also offers nutrition counseling, meal planning, and other services for individual, couples, and family. She's a master at helping you make the mind/body/nutrition connection in a welcoming and accepting setting.

JG: If you can't make it to Jackie's place, she'd be glad to work with you virtually. Visit her website at www.eatingforwellness.net or give her at call directly at 213-822-2634.

JS: We've certainly failed to mention lots of terrific resources in this chapter. If you're one of our paleo friends and we haven't given you a nod, we apologize, and assure our readers it's not because you aren't awesome. There's a growing paleo community out there, and every day it is producing even more talented coaches, insightful writers, brilliant scientists, skilled doctors, and terrific chefs.

JG: And more regular folks like us, who find their paleo Tao and manage to change their lives for the better.

JS: If you know of a great paleo resource that we failed to mention here and you'd like to let the community know about it, visit our website at www.paleotao.com and send us a message. We'd be glad to add your recommendation to the Resources section of our website.

JG: The more the merrier. And buy Joe's book. He gives half the proceeds to charity - and he needs the money. He's been wearing the same underwear for a week now.

JS: I like these. The leopard print is extraordinarily paleo and very flattering.

JG: I guess washing them didn't occur to you.

JS: Not so much.

APPENDIX A: MOVE

JG: I like to move it move it.

JS: Don't. Please.

JG: I like to move it move it.

JS: Jason. The book is over. This is just the workout template section.

JG: Nothing's over till we say it's over!

JS: Oh boy.

JG: Was it over when the Germans bombed Pearl Harbor?

JS: Please. Less shtick, more workout template.

JG: OK. Before we start, we'd like to remind you that this is only one of many acceptable paleo movement templates. Eventually you might end up doing something completely different. Darryl Edwards, for example, uses a template for his clients that may look entirely different. It's up to you to find the Tao that maximizes your health and happiness. That being said, if you're looking for some guidance this is an excellent place to start.

JS: Enough qualifying. Let 'er rip.

JG: Fair enough. We're going to divide this section based on levels of fitness, but these templates are designed to be evolutionary - as you lose fat and improve your fitness level, you can bump up your level of movement.

JS: I see what you did there. Anyway, we'd like to reiterate as well that if you are unfamiliar with any of the exercises we mention, or if you feel that you need professional assistance to start your workout program, hire a professional to help you.

JG: First and foremost, if you are sedentary and/or have very high levels of body fat, we suggest a walking program ONLY for now.

JS: Walk in a LEISURELY manner, either outside or on a treadmill. Do not walk at a pace that requires labored breathing or intensive effort. If you are completely sedentary and significantly overweight, we'd like you to start with a ten minute walk and add a few minutes of duration per week.

JG: At first walk three times a week, gradually adding a walking session until you reach five sessions per week. Eventually, each of these walks should be a minimum of half an hour in duration and a maximum of one hour.

JS: In the chapter *Move* we explained the tremendous health benefits that can be achieved with a walking program alone. However once your Tao has taken you to a point where you feel like you are ready for another element, we suggest adding one sprinting session and one weightlifting session per week.

JG: This doesn't mean that you should stop walking, however. You should continue to take those long, leisurely walks as often as you can.

JS: Right. The first task of your lifting sessions is to get comfortable with proper form. This might mean lifting extremely light weights for quite some time until your form supports higher effort. Eventually, we'd like you to shoot for a minimum 80% of your maximum effort in each set with a target of 95%. Your trainer can help you determine where those numbers are in terms of actual weight.

JG: Your initial lifting schedule should be once weekly, and should incorporate the following:

- A whole body movement like front or back squats, dead lifts, power cleans, or snatch lifts. You should perform a pyramid of sets in the following pattern: 5 repetitions, 3 repetitions, 1 repetition, 3 repetitions, 5 repetitions.

- A partial body movement like standing military or overhead presses, bench presses, or lunges. These should also be performed in a 5, 3, 1, 3, 5 pyramid.

- As your fitness level improves, you can add a fitness/support, movement, such as kettle bell swings, farmer's carries, or Turkish getups. You should perform five sets of five repetitions of the movement you choose at the end of the workout.

JS: You should not huff and puff at all in between these sets. Take adequate recovery time in between in order to allow heartbeat and respiration to return to a resting state. Two minutes minimum is a good starting point.

JG: We can't overemphasize enough that the purpose of this sequence has nothing to do with cardio or breathing hard. You're working your fast twitch muscle fibers and creating a hormonal reaction that will burn fat and build muscle over the next twenty-four hours. I often say that the purpose of the workout isn't the workout.

JS: That's pretty deep there Buddha.

JG: What is the sound of one hand clapping you right in your yap Joe?

JS: Again, it's vital that you consume a significant meal composed of protein AND carbs within an hour of finishing this workout in order to take advantage of the insulin sensitivity you've created and to maximize muscle building and fat loss.

JG: You should also have a day of rest before and after this workout to avoid overtraining. Remember rest doesn't preclude those long, slow walks which you should shoot for even on rest days. You might even want to take one the same day you lift, and that's just fine.

JS: At the same time you add a lifting session you might want to add an interval sprinting session. We recommend it once weekly.

JG: Make sure that you stretch adequately before and after sprints. At first, try for a short, choppy stride instead of a long one in order to avoid hamstring or groin pulls. Find a good pair of shoes too.

JS: I actually prefer Vibram Five Fingers shoes which are minimalist and have almost no support. I don't care about the lawsuit, they are excellent. But find what works best for you. We'd like you to start with eight intervals. You might begin with your sprint as a 50-yard jog followed by a 50-yard walk and a minute of rest.

JG: As your conditioning improves increase the distance and work toward a full-out sprint during the sprinting portion, followed by a brisk walk for the same distance, followed by a short rest.

JS: Eventually you can eliminate rest entirely and up the number of intervals. Be careful, however, because too many sprints or too long a workout duration and you eliminate the benefit and start to do harm. Although you may have a lot of enthusiasm, you have to ease into it.

JG: At my relatively advanced level of fitness, I do ten to twelve intervals, each composed of a 110-meter dead sprint followed by a 110-meter brisk walk with no rest in between. I do them in the cul-de-sac in front of my home or at the local high school track. I often do these sprints barefoot on the

beach while on business trips. Firm sand is an absolutely ideal surface.

JS: If you are unable to sprint outside, you might use a treadmill program where you alternate walking with a fast run. Perform 2 minute intervals comprised of 1 ½ minutes of a comfortable walk followed by 30 of a fast jog. Again, shoot for 8 intervals to start and eventually extend yourself to 10-12, while increasing the run portion to 45 seconds and decreasing the walk to 1 minute 15 seconds.

JG: You need a day off before and a day off after sprinting, and this doesn't exclude walking.

JS: As with the lifting sessions, the sprinting workouts are designed to exercise the fast twitch muscle fibers. This in turn will increase insulin sensitivity, increase muscle, and burn fat. Once again, you'll need to eat within an hour after your sprints in order to maximize the positive effects.

JG: When your level of fitness is such that you can handle a regular schedule of sprinting and lifting along with your walks, you can consider adding high intensity interval training (HIIT) training to your repertoire.

JS: Remember, HIIT training is typically a series of exercises performed in a circuit at relatively high repetitions with minimal or no rest in between stations.

JG: We look at HIIT like dynamite. Used properly, it can be an effective and powerful tool, especially when it comes to burning fat. Used incorrectly, it can blow up in your face in the form of overtraining or even fatigue. It is absolutely critical that you rest the day before and after a HIIT session. Do not attempt to back a HIIT session up to a lifting or a sprinting day.

JS: You need to achieve a basic level of fitness before you start HIIT training and be comfortable with sprints and weights.

JG: HIIT training should be performed no more than once a week. For a basic routine, pick six exercises from the list below:

- Push-ups (set of 8-12)
- Pull-ups (assisted if necessary, set of 5)
- Sit-ups or Swiss ball crunches (set of 10)
- Lunges (weighted or unweighted, set of 10)
- Box or platform jumps (set of 8)
- Kettle bell swings (set of 8)
- Rowing machine sprints (30 seconds)
- Jumping jacks (set of 10-15)
- Jump rope (30 seconds)
- Kettle bell goblet squats (set of 8-12)
- Burpees (set of 8-10)
- Kettle bell Turkish getups (set of 5)
- Wall Squats (set of 8-10)
- Running in place (30 seconds, high knees)
- Incline push-ups (set of 8-12)
- Hyperextensions (set of 8-12)
- Mountain climbers (set of 8-12)

JS: Start with an eight-minute session. Move as quickly as possible between your six selected exercises, taking a short break of 10-15 seconds at the end of each six-movement circuit. Do each exercise at high intensity.

JG: If you're not used to this kind of exercise you're likely to find it exhausting at first. That's why we recommend you start with no more than an eight minute session, extending the total length of the workouts about a minute at a time every few weeks and gradually eliminating the rest period at the end of each circuit.

JS: We'd never advise you to do HIIT more than once per week, or move beyond twenty minute sessions. We want you to work well within the glycolytic pathway - this means that we don't want your body to exhaust glycogen stores and start catabolizing your muscle tissue.

JG: Excessive or overlong HIIT training can also trigger excessive cortisol releases, which we want to avoid.

JS: If you're going to do HIIT training, you need to significantly increase your intake of starchy carbs both the night before your session and during the meal immediately following the workout.

JG: Fuel and refill those glycogen stores. Don't risk bonking during your workouts or jeopardizing your recovery. If fueled properly, HIIT can burn fat off your body like a paleo blowtorch and significantly increase your level of functional fitness.

JS: Let's review. First, if you are sedentary or carry a large amount of body fat, start with a walking program until your fitness level improves significantly. Believe us, it will, if you follow the basic template we've laid out for you. If you go too fast, you can sabotage your progress and it will take much longer to get back on track.

JG: Next, add in a weight session and a sprint workout once each per week, adding intensity as your fitness continues to improve. If you're pretty fit to begin with, you can start at this point.

JS: Finally, if you feel that HIIT training supports your goals, you can add a HIIT session per week - provided you're comfortable with sprinting and weights.

JG: If you choose to follow the template we've provided, you're going to be seriously fit by the time you hit the upper limits we've laid out for you. You're going to feel great. You're also going to be pretty darned lean, because this template is designed to burn fat and increase healthy, lean, muscle. You're going to enjoy what you see in the mirror in the morning too.

JS: Just remember that for us, movement is a means to an end. The idea is to enjoy a happy and healthy life, not to become a gym rat. Don't become obsessed with your workouts. This can lead to addictive behavior that can compromise and eventually ruin your newfound health and vitality. More is not necessarily better - in fact, in this case, it usually isn't.

JG: Think we've just about covered it?

JS: I think we've beaten it to death.

JG: What do you feel like doing now?

JS: Should we go to the gym? There's a two hour marathon Zumba class that starts in twenty minutes.

JG: You haven't paid any attention to anything we've been talking about for this entire chapter, have you?

JS: You're so cute when you're angry.

APPENDIX B: 12-WEEK MEAL PLAN
(recipes for all * items start on page 221)

	Breakfast	Lunch	Dinner
Week 1			
Day 1	Basic Mini Crustless Quiche*	Taco-seasoned lettuce wraps*, Jicama Spears w/ lime, Guacamole	Chicken and Mixed Veggie Stir-fry*
Day 2	Tomato Basil Frittata*, breakfast sausage*	Left over stir fry	Grilled Garlic Flank Steak* (Make extra for salad), Asparagus, Steamed Spinach
Day 3	Eggs scrambled with spinach, bacon, avocado	Steak Salad (leftover flank steak on salad) w/ balsamic dressing*	Crock Pot Chicken*, Bacon Roasted Broccoli*, Cauliflower Rice*
Day 4	Paleo Crunch Cereal*, Berries, Bacon	Leftover Chicken, Left over broccoli, Apple	Shrimp Scampi with Zucchini noodles*
Day 5	Basic Mini Crustless Quiche*	Spaghetti Squash and Meatballs	Bacon Wrapped Chicken*, Green Beans, Sauteed Cabbage
Day 6	Tomato Basil Frittata*, breakfast sausage*	Chicken Fingers*, carrots, cucumbers	Honey Mustard Chicken*, Mixed Veggies, Oven Roasted Sweet Potato Spears
Day 7	Asparagus Ham and Egg Bake*, breakfast sausage*	Taco-seasoned lettuce wraps*, Jicama Spears w/ lime, Guacamole	Khalua Pork* (double), Mashed Sweet Potato, Cabbage Salad

	Breakfast	Lunch	Dinner
Week 2			
Day 1	Paleo Crunch Cereal*, Berries, Bacon	Pulled Khalua pork with bbq sauce stuffed into a sweet potato	Bacon Wrapped Chicken*, Green Beans, Sauteed Cabbage
Day 2	Sweet Potato Muffins*, Bacon	Turkey Club Salad	Burger Bar and Butternut Squash Fries Topping Suggestions: Bacon, avocado, grilled onions, tomato
Day 3	Turkey or Pork Breakfast Sausage*, eggs, Sliced tomatoes	Chicken Fingers*, carrots, cucumbers	Chili* served over cauliflower rice* Salad
Day 4	Tex-Mex Egg Bake*, Orange	Left over Chili and Cauliflower Rice	Pan Fried Cod Spinach sauteed w/butter and garlic Cauli rice pilaf*
Day 5	Eggs scrambled with spinach, bacon, avocado	Ham & Turkey Roll-ups, dill pickles, cherry tomatoes	Meatloaf* Sauteed Cabbage Mashed Sweet Potato
Day 6	Basic Mini Crustless Quiche*	Leftover Meatloaf, Sauteed Cabbage, Mashed Sweet Potato	Teriyaki Chicken* Asian Fried Cauli Rice*
Day 7	Sweet Potato Hash and Eggs*, bacon	Leftover Teriyaki Chicken, Green Salad	Turkey Wings Green Beans Kale

	Breakfast	Lunch	Dinner
Week 3			
Day 1	Bacon and Sweet Potato Bake	Spinach Salad with bacon and Honey Poppy Seed dressing	Maple Chili Chicken* Bacon Roast Broccoli* Shaved Brussels Sprouts
Day 2	Hard Boiled Eggs, Bacon, Apple	leftover maple chili chicken, green salad	Shrimp Scampi with Zucchini noodles*
Day 3	Sweet Potato Hash and Eggs*, bacon	Leftover Spaghetti Squash and Meatballs	Honey Mustard Chicken*, Mixed Veggies, Oven Roasted Sweet Potato Spears
Day 4	Basic Mini Crustless Quiche*	Chopped Leftover Honey mustard chicken over mixed greens with red onion	Burger Bar and Butternut Squash Fries. Topping Suggestions: Bacon, avocado, grilled onions, tomato
Day 5	Bacon and Sweet Potato Bake	Chicken Fingers, carrots, cucumbers	Firecracker Salmon* Garlic Butter Zucchini Noodles Green beans
Day 6	Turkey or Pork Breakfast Sausage*, eggs, Sliced tomatoes	Spinach Salad with bacon and Honey Poppy Seed dressing	Chicken and Mixed Veggie Stir-fry*
Day 7	Scrambled Egg Nests*, breakfast sausage	Leftover Chicken Stir-fry	Crock Pot Chicken*, Bacon Roasted Broccoli*, Cauliflower Rice

	Breakfast	Lunch	Dinner
Week 4			
Day 1	Paleo Crunch Cereal*, Berries, Bacon	Leftover Chicken, left over broccoli	Meatloaf* Sauteed Cabbage Mashed Sweet Potato
Day 2	Eggs scrambled with spinach, bacon, avocado	Taco-seasoned lettuce wraps*, Jicama Spears w/ lime, Guacamole	Pan Fried Cod Spinach sauteed w/butter and garlic Cauli rice pilaf*
Day 3	Bacon and Sweet Potato Bake	Ham & Turkey Roll-ups Dill Pickles Baby Carrots	Turkey Wings Green Beans Kale
Day 4	Basic Mini Crustless Quiche*	Turkey Club Salad	Mongolian Beef* Asian Cauliflower Rice* Stir-fry Veggies
Day 5	Hard Boiled Eggs, Bacon, Apple	leftover Mongolian Beef, stir-fry veggies	Chili* served over cauliflower rice Salad
Day 6	Bacon and Sweet Potato Bake	Leftover Chili over cauliflower rice	Khalua Pork*, Mashed Sweet Potato, Cabbage Salad
Day 7	Paleo Crunch Cereal*, Berries, Bacon	Pulled Khalua pork* with bbq sauce stuffed into a sweet potato	Grilled Garlic Flank Steak* (Make extra for Salad), Asparagus, Steamed Spinach

	Breakfast	Lunch	Dinner
Week 5			
Day 1	Turkey or Pork Breakfast Sausage*, eggs, Sliced tomatoes	Steak Salad	Firecracker Salmon* Garlic Butter Spaghetti Squash Green beans
Day 2	Basic Mini Crustless Quiche*	Spinach Salad with bacon and Honey Poppy Seed dressing	Stuffed Peppers* Squash, Mushrooms and Onions sauteed in butter
Day 3	Tomato Basil Frittata*, breakfast sausage*	Taco-seasoned lettuce wraps*, Jicama Spears w/ lime, Guacamole	Chicken Fajitas, Spanish Cauli Rice*
Day 4	Paleo Crunch Cereal*, Berries, Bacon	Left over chicken fajitas, green salad	Beef stir-fry*, Asian Cauliflower Rice
Day 5	Basic Mini Crustless Quiche*	leftover beef-stir fry	Bacon Wrapped Chicken*, Green Beans, Sauteed Cabbage
Day 6	Tomato Basil Frittata*, breakfast sausage*	leftover bacon wrapped chicken, baby carrots, cherry tomatoes	Chicken Fingers*, sweet potato fries, cabbage salad*
Day 7	Scrambled Egg Nests*, breakfast sausage*	Ham & Turkey Roll-ups, dill pickles, cherry tomatoes	Crock Pot Chicken*, Bacon Roasted Broccoli*, Cauliflower Rice*

	Breakfast	Lunch	Dinner
Week 6			
Day 1	Paleo Crunch Cereal*, Berries, Bacon	Leftover Chicken, left over broccoli	Khalua Pork*, Mashed Sweet Potato, Cabbage Salad
Day 2	Bacon and Sweet Potato Bake	Pulled Khalua pork with bbq sauce stuffed into a sweet potato	Burger Bar and Butternut Squash Fries Topping Suggestions: Bacon, avocado, grilled onions, tomato
Day 3	Eggs scrambled with spinach, bacon, avocado	Turkey Club Salad	Chicken Piccata*, Cauliflower rice Steamed Vegetables,
Day 4	Basic Mini Crustless Quiche*	leftover chicken piccata, cauliflower rice	Pan Fried Cod Spinach sauteed w/butter and garlic
Day 5	Sweet Potato Hash and Eggs*, bacon	Ham & Turkey Roll-ups Dill Pickles Baby Carrots	Cauli rice pilaf* Meatloaf* Sauteed Cabbage Mashed Sweet Potato
Day 6	Bacon and Sweet Potato Bake	Leftover Meatloaf, Sauteed Cabbage, Mashed Sweet Potato	Buffalo Wings, carrots, celery, butternut squash fries
Day 7	Hard Boiled Eggs, Bacon, Apple	Spinach Salad with bacon and Honey Poppy Seed dressing	Teriyaki Chicken* Asian Fried Cauli-Rice*

	Breakfast	Lunch	Dinner
Week 7			
Day 1	Sweet Potato Hash and Eggs*, bacon	Leftover Teriyaki Chicken, Green Salad	Chili* served over cauliflower rice* Salad
Day 2	Basic Mini Crustless Quiche*	Leftover Chili over cauliflower rice	Maple Glazed Chicken* Bacon Roast Broccoli* Shaved Brussels Sprouts
Day 3	Bacon and Sweet Potato Bake	Spinach Salad with bacon and Honey Poppy Seed dressing	Burger Bar and Butternut Squash Fries Topping Suggestions: Bacon, avocado, grilled onions, tomato
Day 4	Turkey or Pork Breakfast Sausage*, eggs, Sliced tomatoes	Spinach Salad with bacon and Honey Poppy Seed dressing	Firecracker Salmon* Garlic Butter Zucchini Noodles Green beans
Day 5	Scrambled Egg Nests*, breakfast sausage	Leftover Spaghetti Squash and Meatballs	Bacon Wrapped Chicken*, Green Beans, Sauteed Cabbage
Day 6	Paleo Crunch Cereal*, Berries, Bacon	Chicken Fingers, carrots, cucumbers	Crock Pot Chicken*, Bacon Roasted Broccoli*, Cauliflower Rice
Day 7	Eggs scrambled with spinach, bacon, avocado	Leftover Chicken, left over broccoli	Honey Mustard Chicken*, Mixed Veggies, Oven Roasted Sweet Potato Spears

	Breakfast	Lunch	Dinner
Week 8			
Day 1	Bacon and Sweet Potato Bake	Chopped Leftover Honey mustard chicken over mixed greens with red onion	Chicken Fajitas, Spanish Cauli Rice
Day 2	Basic Mini Crustless Quiche*	Leftover Chicken Fajitas, green salad	Honey Chicken*, Zucchini noodles, mixed vegetables
Day 3	Hard Boiled Eggs, Bacon, Apple	leftover honey chicken, zucchini noodles	Beef stir-fry*, Asian Cauliflower Rice
Day 4	Bacon and Sweet Potato Bake	leftover beef-stir fry	Meatloaf* Sauteed Cabbage Mashed Sweet Potato
Day 5	Basic Mini Crustless Quiche*	Leftover Meatloaf, Sauteed Cabbage, Mashed Sweet Potato	Chili* served over cauliflower rice Salad
Day 6	Turkey or Pork Breakfast Sausage*, eggs, Sliced tomatoes	Leftover Chili over cauliflower rice	Mongolian Beef* Asian Cauliflower Rice* Stir-fry Veggies
Day 7	Basic Mini Crustless Quiche*	leftover Mongolian Beef, stir-fry veggies	Honey Chicken*, Zucchini noodles, mixed vegetables

	Breakfast	Lunch	Dinner
Week 9			
Day 1	Paleo Crunch Cereal*, Berries, Bacon	leftover honey chicken, zucchini noodles	Khalua Pork*, Mashed Sweet Potato, Cabbage Salad
Day 2	Eggs scrambled with spinach, bacon, avocado	Pulled Khalua pork with bbq sauce stuffed into a sweet potato	Grilled Garlic Flank Steak*, Asparagus, Steamed Spinach
Day 3	Sweet Potato Muffins*, Bacon	Steak Salad	Pan Fried Cod Spinach sauteed w/butter and garlic Cauli rice pilaf*
Day 4	Turkey or Pork Breakfast Sausage*, eggs, Sliced tomatoes	Spinach Salad with bacon and Honey Poppy Seed dressing	Bacon Wrapped Chicken*, Green Beans, Sauteed Cabbage
Day 5	Basic Mini Crustless Quiche*	Taco Boats*, Jicama Spears w/ lime, Guacamole	Chicken Piccata*, Cauliflower rice Steamed Vegetables,
Day 6	Tomato Basil Frittata*, breakfast sausage*	leftover chicken piccata, cauliflower rice, steamed vegetables	Chicken Fajitas, Spanish Cauli Rice*
Day 7	Eggs scrambled with spinach, bacon, avocado	leftover chicken fajitas over mixed greens	Crock Pot Chicken*, Bacon Roasted Broccoli*, Cauliflower Rice*

	Breakfast	Lunch	Dinner
Week 10			
Day 1	Basic Mini Crustless Quiche*	Leftover Chicken, Left over broccoli, Apple	Bacon Wrapped Chicken*, Green Beans, Sauteed Cabbage
Day 2	Tomato Basil Frittata*, breakfast sausage*	Ham and Turkey roll-ups, dill pickles, baby carrots, cherry tomatoes	Khalua Pork*, Mashed Sweet Potato, Cabbage Salad
Day 3	Scrambled Egg Nests*, breakfast sausage*	Pulled Khalua pork with bbq sauce stuffed into a sweet potato	Honey Mustard Chicken*, Mixed Veggies, Oven Roasted Sweet Potato Spears
Day 4	Paleo Crunch Cereal*, Berries, Bacon	leftover honey mustard chicken on mixed greens with honey mustard dressing	Burger Bar and Butternut Squash Fries Topping Suggestions: Bacon, avocado, grilled onions, tomato
Day 5	Tex Mex Bake*, Sliced Jicama	Chicken Fingers*, carrots, cucumbers	Chicken Piccata*, Cauliflower rice Steamed Vegetables,
Day 6	Eggs scrambled with spinach, bacon, avocado	leftover chicken piccata, cauliflower rice, steamed vegetables	Beef stir-fry*, Asian Cauliflower Rice
Day 7	Sweet Potato Hash and Eggs*, bacon	leftover beef stir-fry	Pan Fried Cod Spinach sauteed w/butter and garlic Cauli rice pilaf*

	Breakfast	Lunch	Dinner
Week 11			
Day 1	Bacon and Sweet Potato Bake	Taco-seasoned lettuce wraps*, Jicama Spears w/ lime, Guacamole	Chili* served over cauliflower rice* Salad
Day 2	Sweet Potato Hash and Eggs*, bacon	Left over Chili and Cauliflower Rice	Meatloaf* Sauteed Cabbage Mashed Sweet Potato
Day 3	Basic Mini Crustless Quiche*	Leftover Meatloaf, Sauteed Cabbage, Mashed Sweet Potato	Buffalo Wings, carrots, celery, butternut squash fries
Day 4	Bacon and Sweet Potato Bake	Turkey Club Salad	Turkey Wings Green Beans Kale
Day 5	Turkey or Pork Breakfast Sausage*, eggs, Sliced tomatoes	Spinach Salad with bacon and Honey Poppy Seed dressing	Burger Bar and Butternut Squash Fries Topping Suggestions: Bacon, avocado, grilled onions, tomato
Day 6	Scrambled Egg Nests*, breakfast sausage	Chicken Fingers, carrots, cucumbers	Shrimp Scampi with Zucchini noodles*
Day 7	Paleo Crunch Cereal*, Berries, Bacon	Leftover Spaghetti Squash and Meatballs	Honey Mustard Chicken*, Mixed Veggies, Oven Roasted Sweet Potato Spears

	Breakfast	Lunch	Dinner
Week 12			
Day 1	Eggs scrambled with spinach, bacon, avocado	Chopped Leftover Honey mustard chicken over mixed greens with red onion	Honey Chicken*, Zucchini noodles, mixed vegetables
Day 2	Bacon and Sweet Potato Bake	leftover honey chicken, zucchini noodles	Firecracker Salmon* Garlic Butter Zucchini Noodles Green beans
Day 3	Basic Mini Crustless Quiche*	Spinach Salad with bacon and Honey Poppy Seed dressing	Bacon Wrapped Chicken*, Green Beans, Sauteed Cabbage
Day 4	Hard Boiled Eggs, Bacon, Apple	leftover bacon wrapped chicken, baby carrots, cherry tomatoes	Crock Pot Chicken*, Bacon Roasted Broccoli*, Cauliflower Rice
Day 5	Bacon and Sweet Potato Bake	Leftover Chicken, left over broccoli	Meatloaf* Sauteed Cabbage Mashed Sweet Potato
Day 6	Paleo Crunch Cereal*, Berries, Bacon	Leftover Meatloaf, Sauteed Cabbage, Mashed Sweet Potato	Pan Fried Cod Spinach sauteed w/butter and garlic Cauli rice pilaf*
Day 7	Turkey or Pork Breakfast Sausage*, eggs, Sliced tomatoes	Ham & Turkey Roll-ups Dill Pickles Baby Carrots	Turkey Wings Green Beans Kale

APPENDIX C:
RECIPES (ALPHABETICAL), TIPS AND TRICKS, SALAD DRESSING MATRIX

Asparagus Ham and Egg Bake

Ingredients:
1 ½ cups cooked ham, chopped
1 pound fresh asparagus spears, cut into 1-inch pieces
4 cups sweet potatoes, shredded
1 medium onion, chopped
12 eggs
1 cup full-fat coconut milk
1 tablespoon lemon juice
1 teaspoon pepper
1 teaspoon sea salt
2 teaspoons ground mustard
1 cup roughly crushed pork rinds
2 tablespoons butter/ghee

Directions:
Prepare a 13x9-inch glass baking dish with butter/ghee, set aside. In large bowl, toss ham, asparagus, sweet potatoes, and onion. Spoon into baking dish. In same bowl, beat eggs, milk, lemon, pepper, sea salt and mustard until well mixed. Pour egg mixture over potato mixture. Cover, refrigerate 8 hours or overnight (optional). Heat oven to 325 degrees. Bake, uncovered, for 35 minutes. Sprinkle pork rinds partially baked casserole. Bake uncovered 30 to 35 minutes longer or until knife inserted in center comes out clean. Remove from oven and let stand 15 minutes before serving.

Bacon and Sweet Potato Bake
*Can be made the night before

Ingredients:
½ pound bacon, cut into 1-inch pieces
1 small onion, chopped
1 red bell pepper, chopped
½ cup fresh mushrooms, sliced
1 tablespoon Dijon mustard
½ teaspoon sea sea salt
½ teaspoon pepper
6 eggs
2 cups shredded sweet potato
1 tablespoon butter/ghee

Directions:
Prepare 13x9 inch baking dish with butter/ghee taking care to cover all surfaces then set aside. In skillet, cook bacon until crisp, then, using slotted spoon, remove from pan to small bowl. Reserve about 2 tablespoons of the drippings in the pan.

Over medium heat, add onion, bell pepper and mushrooms and cook 5 minutes, stirring occasionally. Stir in mustard, sea salt and pepper. In large bowl, beat eggs then set aside.

Spread half of shredded sweet potato in prepared baking dish. Spread onion mixture evenly on top. Spread remaining hash browns over top. Pour egg mixture on top. Cover; refrigerate 8 hours or overnight.

Heat oven to 325 degrees. Uncover; bake 50 to 60 minutes. Sprinkle with remaining bacon. Bake 3 to 5 minutes longer or until knife inserted in center comes out clean.

Bacon Roasted Broccoli

Ingredients:
1 pound broccoli florets
5 peeled cloves of garlic
4 slices of bacon cut into bite-size pieces
½ cup avocado oil (can use melted ghee or melted lard)
Sea salt and pepper

Directions:
Preheat oven to 400 degrees. Place the broccoli, bacon, and garlic cloves in a gallon-sized ziploc bag. Add oil and along with a generous amount of salt and freshly ground black pepper. Seal the bag and shake it vigorously. Pour the contents on a foil lined baking tray taking care to make sure that they are in a single layer. Roast the broccoli for 30-35 minutes, rotating the tray and flipping the contents every 10 minutes or so.

Bacon Wrapped Chicken

Ingredients:
1 pound boneless, skinless chicken (can use thighs or breast)
Miss O's salt seasoning (see *Tips and Tricks* section, below)
6-8 strips of bacon

Directions:
Flatten chicken to ½ inch thickness and sprinkle with seasoned salt; roll up. Wrap each with bacon strip. Place, seam side down in a greased 13 x 9 inch baking pan. Bake, uncovered, at 400 degrees for 35-40 minutes or until a thermometer reads 170 degrees. Broil 6 inches from the heat for 5 minutes or until bacon is crisp.

Basic Mini-Crustless Quiche
*Note: A silicone muffin tin works very well for this recipe

Ingredients
1 pound ground pork breakfast sausage (pasture-raised, organic if possible)
1 dozen eggs
1 cup chopped vegetables of choice
Coconut oil or other fat of choice
salt and pepper to taste

Directions
Preheat oven to 350 degrees. Crumble and brown the pork sausage in a frying pan or cast iron skillet. Sauté vegetables in fat for 5 minutes. In a medium/large bowl scramble one dozen large eggs and season with salt and pepper. Add vegetables and cheese to scrambled eggs. Grease the cups of one muffin tin with oil. Place equal amounts of browned sausage in the bottoms of the muffin tins. Pour the scrambled eggs evenly on top of the sausage. The mixture will come almost to the top of the tin. Cook for 20 minutes. Remove from the oven and allow to cool for about 5 minutes. Use a knife to loosen the egg muffin from the sides of the pan.

Basic Stir Fry

Ingredients:
2 pounds of meat, sliced (beef, pork, chicken)
1 clove garlic, minced
2 cups broccoli florets
1 onion, chopped
1 red bell pepper, chopped
2 carrots, chopped
3 tablespoons avocado oil

Sauce:
½ cup organic chicken broth
½ cup coconut aminos (can use tamari)
4 teaspoons rice wine vinegar
4 teaspoons toasted sesame oil
2 teaspoons hot red pepper flakes (optional)
2 teaspoons honey

Directions:
In a large skillet, heat the oils over medium-high heat. Add the meat and cook for 4 to 5 minutes or until lightly browned. Add vegetables and cook an additional 5 minutes, stirring frequently. In a small bowl, combine all sauce ingredients. Add to chicken mixture and bring to a boil over medium-high heat. Reduce heat to medium to medium-low, and simmer for 4 to 5 minutes, or until sauce thickens.

Breakfast Sausage (Turkey)

Ingredients:
1 small onion, diced
1 medium Fuji or Gala apple, peeled and diced
1 pound ground turkey
1 tablespoon sage
1 tablespoon coconut (palm) sugar
½ teaspoon fennel seed
1 teaspoon sea salt
¼ teaspoon freshly ground pepper
2 tablespoons bacon fat (or lard)

Directions
In a large skillet over medium heat, melt fat. Add onion and cook until just translucent, about 2 minutes. Add apples and cook, stirring, 2 more minutes then transfer to a large bowl and cool for 5 minutes. Add remaining ingredients to the bowl with the apples and onions. Gently mix to combine. Heat skillet over medium heat, then using a ⅓ cup measure, scoop then flatten the patties. Cook until the patties are browned and cooked through, about 3 minutes per side, adjusting the heat as necessary to prevent burning.

Cabbage Salad

Ingredients:
1 teaspoon sesame oil

⅓ cup sliced almonds
1 head cabbage, finely chopped
6 green onions, sliced thin

⅔ cup olive oil
2 tablespoons water
¼ cup apple cider vinegar
1 tablespoon raw honey
½ tablespoon organic chicken base
salt and pepper

Directions:
Toast almonds in a skillet on the stove about 10 minutes until lightly toasted. Watch carefully, they can burn quickly. Mix cabbage and green onions in a large bowl. In a separate bowl, whisk oil, water, and vinegar in a bowl. Add honey and chicken base. Pour on dressing and toss well. Add almonds just before serving. Serve immediately.

Cauliflower Rice

Ingredients:

⅓ pound cauliflower
2 tablespoons butter/ghee
1 teaspoon sea salt
½ teaspoon pepper
1 clove garlic, minced

Directions:
Remove the stem and leaves from cauliflower. Cut off florets then place in food processor (or blender then cover with water). Pulse until rice-like consistency (if using a blender, strain into a colander). Melt butter/ghee in medium sized skillet over medium-heat. Add garlic and sauté until fragrant. Add cauli rice and continue to cook for 5-7 minutes or until cauliflower begins to soften.

VARIATIONS: Asian Cauli Rice
Ingredients:
2 tablespoons tamari
2 green onions
¼ cup shredded carrots
1 teaspoon coconut oil
1 scrambled egg

Add onions and carrots at Step 5 above (with garlic). Add scrambled egg, oil, and tamari at Step 6 (with cauli rice).

Cauli Rice Pilaf
¼ cup shredded carrots
1 onion, chopped
1 red bell pepper, chopped
2 tablespoons dried parsley
¼ cup chicken broth

Add vegetables and parsley at Step 5 above.
Add chicken broth at Step 6

Chicken Fajitas

Ingredients:
1 ½ pounds meat (chicken or beef), cut into ¼ inch strips
1 green bell pepper, sliced
1 red bell pepper, sliced
1 onion, sliced

Chicken fajita seasoning:
1 tablespoon chili powder
1 tablespoon salt
½ tablespoon paprika
1 teaspoon onion powder
½ teaspoon garlic powder
½ teaspoon cayenne pepper
¼ teaspoon crushed red pepper flakes
½ teaspoon cumin

Directions: In a medium bowl, mix the seasoning ingredients together. Set aside for later. Sprinkle chicken with seasoning. Add oil to pan then sauté chicken until cooked through. Add veggies and continue cooking until heated through.

Chicken Fingers

Ingredients:
2 pounds boneless, skinless chicken breast tenders
1 cup tapioca starch
½ cup arrowroot
2 tablespoons Miss O's seasoned salt (see Tips and Tricks, below) separated
Lard, tallow or coconut oil for frying

Directions:
In a bowl, season chicken with 1 tablespoon of seasoning
In ziploc bag, combine tapioca, arrowroot and remaining seasoning. Working in small batches, place pieces in bag with tapioca mixture, seal and shake to coat pieces. Remove pieces from tapioca mixture, shaking off excess then fry for 7-10 minutes. Place nuggets on cooling rack in a warm oven to keep them crispy until all batches are finished cooking.

Chicken Piccata

Ingredients:
5 boneless skinless chicken breasts, butterflied
salt and pepper, to taste
½ cup arrowroot
6 tablespoons avocado oil, divided
1 cup chicken broth
3 tablespoons capers, drained and rinsed
1 lemon, juiced
1 tablespoon dried parsley

Directions:
Butterfly each chicken breast and split in half. Season the breasts
with salt and pepper. Dredge each breast in arrowroot and
shake off excess. In a large skillet, heat half of the avocado oil.
Add half of the breasts into the pan and brown 3 minutes per
side. Remove the breasts, add the remaining avocado oil, and
add the other half of the breasts. Brown 3 minutes per side,
remove, and keep warm with the first half of the breasts. Pour
chicken broth into skillet to de-glaze the pan. Bring to a boil,
reduce heat, and simmer until the liquid reduces by half. Add in
capers and lemon juice; bring to a simmer. Add back in chicken
breasts and flip to coat with sauce. Cover and simmer for 5-7
minutes; until the sauce is slightly thickened. Serve topped with
parsley.

Chicken and Mixed Veggie Stir Fry

1 pound boneless skinless chicken breast, sliced
2 tablespoons coconut oil
1 cup each: sliced onion, string beans, chopped broccoli, sliced red bell pepper
1 tablespoon sesame seeds
2 scallions, chopped
Stir-fry sauce
2 tablespoons tamari or coconut aminos
2 tablespoons water
2 cloves garlic, chopped
¼ teaspoon dried ginger

Melt oil in a large skillet over medium-high heat
Add chicken to skillet and cook through, about 5-7 minutes then remove chicken and set aside. While meat cooks, combine sauce ingredients, mix well and set aside. Add all veggies except scallions to pan and cook until tender, about 5 minutes. Add meat back to the pan then add sauce and heat through. Plate and top with sesame seeds and scallions.

Chili

Ingredients:
1 pound Italian sausage
1 pound grass-fed ground beef
3 cans diced fire roasted tomatoes
1 can tomato paste
1 can green chilies
1 cup chicken broth
1 medium onion diced
2 stalks celery diced
2 cloves garlic
2 tablespoons avocado oil
2 tablespoons cumin
1 tablespoon chili powder
Cayenne pepper to taste
Salt and pepper to taste

Directions:
Add avocado oil to pan. Add diced onion, celery and garlic to pan. Sauté 3 minutes until fragrant. Add sausage, ground beef, salt and pepper to pan. Cook through then add tomato paste, tomatoes, chilies, chicken broth and spices. Simmer for 15 minutes then enjoy!!

Crockpot: Brown sausage and ground beef. Add meat and all remaining ingredients to crock pot. Cook on low for 3-4 hours.

Chipotle Meatballs (makes 15-20 meatballs)

Ingredients:
1.8 pounds ground grass-fed beef
3 medium dried chipotle chilies (tinned chipotle can also be used), seeds out
2 tablespoons chopped fresh coriander (cilantro)
2 large garlic cloves, finally diced
1 teaspoon ground coriander seed or powder
1 teaspoon ground cumin seed or powder
1 teaspoon sweet or medium paprika
1 tablespoon avocado oil
1 ½ teaspoon of sea salt
2 tablespoons lard or ghee

Sauce:
½ onion, diced
2 garlic cloves, finely chopped
2 medium chipotle chilies, seeds out (hydrate them in water for an hour if they are dried)
½ teaspoon ground coriander seed
1 teaspoon ground cumin seed or powder
½ teaspoon paprika
2 bay leaves
1 ½ cups diced tomatoes or tomato puree
½ teaspoon sea salt

Directions:
First, sauté onion in lard or ghee for 3-5 minutes, until translucent. While onion is cooking, pre-chop all other ingredients for the meatballs. Slice the chipotle chilies in half and remove the seeds. Chop into small pieces. Combine beef with half of the cooked onion, chopped garlic and chilies, paprika, cumin, coriander seed, salt and avocado oil. Use your hands to combine/mash all of the ingredients into sticky meat dough. Wash your hands and roll the mix into small balls. Set aside on a chopping board until ready to cook. Preheat lard in the large frying pan until sizzling. Add the meatballs and cook

on medium/high heat for 3 minutes on each side or until well-browned. They don't need to be completely cooked yet because we will be adding the sauce and cooking further.

Add the sauce ingredients: the rest of the cooked onion, garlic, the other two chopped chilies and spices. Stir through and then add the tomato puree. Combine and cook for 8-10 minutes uncovered and stir frequently to make sure the meatballs finish cooking evenly and the sauce is well mixed in.

Cinnamon Coconut Flour Pancakes

Ingredients:
4 eggs
1 cup coconut milk
1 tablespoon vanilla extract
1 tablespoon maple syrup
1 tablespoon cinnamon
½ cup coconut flour
½ teaspoon sea salt
1 teaspoon baking soda
Coconut oil for frying

Directions:
In a small bowl beat eggs then mix in remaining wet ingredients. In a medium-sized bowl whisk together dry ingredients. Stir wet mixture into dry until everything is incorporated. Melt coconut oil in a skillet over medium heat. Spoon batter into pan then spread out slightly with the back of the spoon. The pancakes should be 2-3 inches in diameter and about an inch thick. Cook for a 2-3 minutes on each side, until the tops dry out slightly and the bottoms start to brown.

Crock Pot Chicken

Ingredients:
1 whole 3-4 pound chicken
1 tablespoon Miss O's seasoned salt (see Tips and Tricks, below)
2 tablespoons butter/ghee, softened

Directions:
In a small bowl, combine the butter and the seasoned salt. Set aside. Rinse chicken and dry with paper towels. Rub the chicken, inside and out, with the butter/ghee mixture. Put the whole chicken in a 4 quart crockpot, cover and cook for 6-8 hours on low until chicken is tender and thoroughly cooked.

Firecracker Salmon

Ingredients:
8 (4-ounce) salmon fillets
½ cup avocado oil
¼ cup tamari
¼ cup balsamic vinegar
¼ cup green onions, chopped
2 tablespoons honey
2 garlic cloves, minced
1 ½ teaspoons ground ginger
2 teaspoons crushed red pepper flakes
½ teaspoon salt
¼ teaspoon pepper

Directions:
Whisk together all ingredients except filets in medium bowl.
Place filets in a glass baking dish, cover with marinade, cover,
and refrigerate 4 to 6 hours. Preheat broiler to high and broil for
3-4 minutes each side or until fish flakes easily with a fork.

Garlic Flank Steak

Ingredients:
¼ cup balsamic vinegar
¼ cup avocado oil
2 large cloves garlic
1 teaspoon thyme leaves
One 2 ½ pound flank steak
Salt and freshly-ground pepper

Directions
In a blender or food processor, combine the vinegar, oil, garlic and thyme and puree until smooth. In a large glass or ceramic dish, pour the marinade over the steak. Let stand for 15 minutes or more. Heat a grill pan (or prepare broiler). Season the steak with salt and pepper. Grill over moderately high heat, turning once, until medium, about 8 minutes per side. Transfer the steak to a board and let stand for 10 minutes. Slice the steak, transfer to plates and serve.

Honey Chicken

Ingredients:
¼ cup avocado oil

⅓ cup honey

⅓ cup coconut aminos
¼ teaspoon ground black pepper

8 skinless, boneless chicken breast halves, cut into 1″ cubes
2 cloves
5 small onions, cut into 2-inch pieces
2 red bell peppers, cut into 2-inch pieces

Directions:
In a large bowl, whisk together oil, honey, soy sauce and black pepper. Add chicken, garlic, onions and peppers into the bowl, cover and marinade in the refrigerator at least 30 minutes. Heat a skillet over medium heat. Drain chicken and vegetables. Cook for 12-15 minutes, until chicken juices run clear.

Honey Mustard Chicken Thighs

Ingredients:

⅓ cup honey

⅓ cup Dijon mustard
1 clove garlic
2 tablespoons avocado oil
1 teaspoon parsley
1 teaspoon salt
½ teaspoon pepper
2 pounds boneless, skinless, chicken thighs

Directions:
Combine all ingredients, except chicken. Pour over chicken taking care to coat completely. Place in a baking dish in a single layer. Broil high 20-25 minutes turning half way through.

Kahlua Pork

Ingredients:
1 (6 pound) pork butt or shoulder roast
1 ½ tablespoons Hawaiian sea salt
1 tablespoon liquid smoke flavoring

Directions:
Pierce pork all over with a carving fork. Rub salt then liquid smoke over meat. Place roast in a slow cooker. Cover, and cook on low for 3 hours per pound of pork. Remove meat from slow cooker, and shred, adding drippings as needed to moisten.

BBQ Sauce:
Puree the following:
1 onion, minced
2 cloves garlic, minced
1 can (6 oz) tomato paste
1 small can (14oz) crushed tomatoes
¼ cup date paste
½ cup unsweetened applesauce
¼ cup balsamic vinegar
¼ cup white wine vinegar
3 tablespoons organic Dijon mustard
Juice of one lime
2 tablespoons coconut aminos
2-3 tablespoons fresh ginger, grated
¼ teaspoon ground cloves
½ teaspoon ground cinnamon
1 teaspoon smoked paprika
3-4 dried chipotle peppers, chopped
1 cup water

Boil in a saucepan, then simmer on low for 50 minutes.

Maple Chili Chicken

Ingredients:
1 ½ pounds boneless skinless chicken
1 tablespoon chili powder
½ teaspoon salt
½ cup pure maple syrup

Directions:
Pre-heat oven to 350 degrees. Place all ingredients into a large baking dish, turn chicken to coat. Bake until chicken juices run clear about 30-45 minutes.

Meat Loaf

Ingredients:
1 medium onion
1 carrot
1 bell pepper
1 clove garlic
½ pound ground beef
½ pound ground turkey
1 egg
1 cup crushed pork rinds (should resemble bread crumbs)
1 teaspoon smoked paprika
1 tablespoon salt
1 teaspoon pepper

Directions:
Place onion, carrot, bell pepper and garlic in food processor. Pulse until all vegetables are finely chopped. Add veggies to bowl with ground meats, egg, salt, pepper and paprika. Add pork rinds and mix well. Place in loaf pan (or muffin tin to make meat muffins) and bake at 350 degrees for 30-40 minutes. Top with tomato sauce (recipe below).

Mongolian Beef

Ingredients:
2 tablespoons avocado oil
½ teaspoon ginger, minced
1 tablespoon garlic, chopped
½ cup tamari
½ cup water
2 tablespoons molasses
¼ cup coconut sugar
1 pound flank steak, thinly sliced
1 tablespoon arrowroot
4 green onions, chopped
1 teaspoon red pepper flakes (optional)

Directions:
Dissolve coconut sugar in the tamari and the arrowroot into the water. Heat 2 teaspoon of oil in a medium saucepan over medium/low heat. Add ginger, green onions and garlic to the pan. Add beef and brown for 1-2 minutes. Add the tamari with coconut sugar, molasses, and water with arrowroot. Increase the heat to medium and boil the sauce for 2-3 minutes or until the sauce thickens. Remove it from the heat. Sprinkle with red pepper flakes if you like.

Paleo Crunch Cereal (or granola)

Ingredients:
1 cup almond meal
1 cup chopped almonds
1 cup flax meal
½ cup coconut flour
4 tablespoons coconut oil
2 tablespoons maple syrup
4 tablespoons raw honey
2 teaspoons vanilla
2 teaspoons cinnamon
1 teaspoon nutmeg
1 teaspoon salt
½ cup finely chopped dates
2 egg whites

Directions:
Preheat oven to 275. Combine almond meal, flax meal, coconut flour, cinnamon, nutmeg, salt and chopped almonds. In a separate bowl, combine coconut oil, egg whites, maple syrup, raw honey, vanilla and chopped dates. Add coconut oil mixture to almond meal mixture. Thoroughly combine taking care not to break down larger 'nuggets'. Spread mixture on ungreased baking sheet. Bake for 90 minutes stirring every 30 minutes. Cool and store in an airtight container.

Scrambled Egg Nests

Ingredients:
3 cup shredded sweet potatoes
¼ cup tapioca flour (starch)

⅓ cup butter/ghee
½ teaspoon sea salt
¼ teaspoon pepper
6 eggs
½ cup onions, diced

⅓ cup bell peppers, diced
¾ cup breakfast sausage, cooked and chopped

Directions:
Preheat oven to 400 degrees. In a large bowl, toss together the potatoes, tapioca starch, ¼ cup of the butter/ghee, sea salt, and pepper. Spoon ⅓ cup of the potato mixture into each cup of a 12-serving muffin tin. Press the mixture into the bottom and up the sides of each cup, then bake until golden brown, about 30 to 35 minutes.

Remove the nests from the oven and allow them to cool. Meanwhile, whisk together the eggs. Heat a large nonstick sauté pan over medium-high heat then add the remaining butter/ghee to the pan and heat. Add the onions and peppers to the pan and sauté until both are soft and the onions are transparent, about 2 to 3 minutes. Add the sausage and cook until heated through. Add the eggs and stir until the eggs have set. Season with sea salt and pepper to taste.

Remove the potato nests from the muffin tin and place them on an ovenproof platter or cookie sheet. Fill each cup with some of the egg mixture and serve warm.

Shrimp Scampi with Zucchini noodles

Ingredients:
5 medium-sized zucchini
1 ½ pound jumbo shrimp, shelled and deveined
Kosher salt and freshly ground black pepper
2 tablespoons butter/ghee
2 cloves garlic, minced
¼ cup dry white vermouth
1 tablespoon freshly squeezed lemon juice
2 teaspoons flat parsley, finely chopped
¼ teaspoon lemon zest grated

Directions:
Peel and julienne zucchini. Place in colander and sprinkle with 1 tablespoon of the salt. Let sit for 20 minutes then squeeze moisture from noodles. Place noodles in paper towel and squeeze - then pat dry place in bowl. DO NOT SKIP THIS STEP! (unless you want watery noodles).

While zucchini is sweating, put the shrimp on a large pie pan or plate and pat them completely dry with a paper towel. Heat a large skillet over medium heat. Season the shrimp with salt and pepper. Add the butter/ghee to the skillet. Cook the shrimp, in one layer, without moving them, for 1 minute. Add the garlic and cook for 1 minute. Turn the shrimp over and cook for 2 minutes more. Transfer the shrimp to the noodle bowl.

Return the skillet to the heat and pour in the vermouth and lemon juice. Boil the liquid until slightly thickened, about 30 seconds. Scrape up any browned bits from the bottom of the pan with a wooden spoon. Stir the zest and parsley into the sauce. Pour the sauce over the shrimp and noodles, season with salt and pepper to taste and toss to combine. Divide the shrimp among 4 plates or arrange on a platter and serve.

Stuffed peppers

Ingredients:
8 bell peppers
1 pound Italian sausage (gluten and hormone-free)
1 pound grass-fed ground beef
1 onion, chopped
2 cloves garlic, minced
½ cup mushrooms, chopped
1 head of cauliflower, riced
2 tablespoons tomato paste
1 teaspoon sea salt
½ teaspoon pepper

Directions:
Preheat oven to 350. Clean and remove the tops of the bell peppers, removing internal membrane. Brown sausage and beef in a large pan over medium heat adding salt and pepper then remove and set aside. In the same skillet add garlic, mushrooms and onions scraping up browned meat bits. Mix in cauliflower and sauté for about 3 minutes. Add tomato paste and meat back in mixing well. Stuff peppers with about 2-3 tablespoons of the meat mixture then place in 8×12 inch pan. Cover loosely with foil and bake for 30 minutes.

Sweet Potato Hash and Eggs

Ingredients:
4 slices thick-cut bacon, cut in 1-inch pieces
4 sweet potatoes, peeled, finely chopped
1 cup chopped onions (2 medium)
½ cup green bell pepper, chopped
½ cup red bell pepper, chopped
½ teaspoon sea salt
¼ teaspoon pepper
2 teaspoons thyme
2 tablespoons parsley
4 eggs

Directions:
In skillet, cook bacon over medium heat about 5 minutes or until crisp. Remove bacon from skillet and set aside. To drippings in skillet, add sweet potatoes, onions and bell peppers. Cook about 20 minutes, stirring occasionally, until potatoes are tender and onions and peppers have browned. Sprinkle potato mixture with sea salt and pepper. Return bacon to skillet. Stir in thyme and parsley. Add fried eggs to top of hash.

Sweet Potato Muffins (makes 4 muffins)

1 large sweet potato
1 egg
1 ½ teaspoon minced dried onion
1 bunch chives
1 teaspoon coconut oil
Sea salt to taste

Preheat oven to 400 degrees. Grate the sweet potato and combine with the egg, mixing thoroughly. Grease the muffin tray with coconut oil. Fill the bacon cup with the grated potato mix and sprinkle with the minced dried onion. Add sea salt to taste. Bake for 45 minutes.

Taco-seasoned lettuce wraps (Taco Seasoning)

Ingredients:
2 ½ tablespoons chili powder
1 ½ tablespoons paprika
2 tablespoons cumin,
2 teaspoons oregano,
1 tablespoon garlic powder
1 tablespoon onion powder
½ teaspoon cayenne pepper (optional/to taste)
2 teaspoons sea salt

Directions:
Combine all ingredients. Store in airtight container. Use 2
tablespoons for every pound of browned ground meat.

Serve wrapped in iceberg lettuce leaves.

Teriyaki Chicken

Ingredients:
4 boneless skinless chicken pieces
1 clove garlic
½ cup honey
1 cup tamari
¼ cup water
¼ teaspoon pepper
1 ½ teaspoon ground ginger
¼ cup white wine

Directions:
In a bowl, combine marinade ingredients. Place chicken in freezer bag. Pour marinade over chicken, seal bag, and let marinate at least an hour. Remove chicken from marinade. Grill chicken until juices run clear, occasionally brushing with marinade.

Tex-Mex Egg Bake
(Can be made the night before)

Ingredients:
12 oz bulk spicy pork sausage (gluten-free)
4 cup shredded sweet potato
1 onion, chopped
1 4.5 oz can chopped green chiles, undrained
6 eggs
½ cup almond milk
¼ teaspoon sea salt
1 cup salsa
1 tablespoon lard/bacon fat/ghee

Directions:
Coat 13x9 inch glass baking dish with fat of choice. In 10-inch skillet, cook sausage over medium heat 8 to 10 minutes, stirring occasionally, until no longer pink. Drain on paper towel.

Spread sweet potatoes in prepared baking dish then sprinkle with sausage and green chiles. In medium bowl, beat eggs, almond milk and sea salt until well blended. Pour over sweet potato mixture. Cover and refrigerate at least 8 hours but no longer than 12 hours.

Heat oven to 350 degrees. Bake uncovered 50 to 60 minutes or until knife inserted near center comes out clean. Let stand 10 minutes. Cut into squares. Serve with salsa.

Tomato Basil Frittata

Ingredients:
6 large eggs
¼ cup almond milk
2 tablespoons avocado oil
2 large ripe tomatoes, peeled and sliced
1 Tablespoon slivered basil leaves
Sea salt and freshly ground black pepper

Directions
Preheat the broiler. In a large bowl, beat the eggs with the milk. In a large cast-iron skillet, heat oil over medium heat. Pour in the egg mixture then scatter the tomatoes and basil over the eggs. Season with sea salt and pepper to taste. When the bottom just begins to brown, place the skillet under the broiler for about 2 minutes or just until the top is set. Remove from the oven and use a large spatula to transfer the frittata to a serving platter. Cool about 10 minutes, cut into wedges, and serve.

TIPS AND TRICKS

Burger Bar - A grass-fed hamburger patty and all of your favorite toppings!

Buffalo Wings - Chicken wings, fried naked in lard (or other fat of choice) and the hottest sauce that you can stand.

Steamed Spinach - In a steamer, cook 1 pound spinach for 3 to 5 minutes or until tender. Add butter/ghee and garlic for extra flavor.

Ham & Turkey Roll-ups - 1 slice of ham, 1 slice of turkey rolled around a pickle; Add mustard for extra zing!

Shaved Brussels sprouts - Brussels sprouts, trimmed, sliced thin using a mandolin or sharp knife.

Mashed Sweet Potato - bake in a 350 degree oven until soft then let cool, peel and mash with a potato masher. Add butter/ghee and cinnamon for extra flavor.

Pan Fried Cod - Salt and pepper both sides of cod fillets that have been patted dry. Add fat of choice to skillet over medium heat; fry until fish flakes easily with a fork – about 3-4 minutes per side.

Jicama Spears w/lime - peel and slice jicama into spears; squeeze fresh lime over spears. Add chili powder for extra kick.

Guacamole - 1 avocado (mashed) , ¼ teaspoon salt, 2 tablespoon salsa, ½ teaspoon garlic powder, ½ teaspoon lime juice; combine all ingredients.

Turkey Club Salad - meat (usually turkey, chicken, and bacon), tomato, lettuce, and dressing of choice.

Turkey Wings - season wings, place in crock-pot on low for 4-5 hours or in 350 degree oven for 45 minutes.

Tomato Sauce:
1 15 oz can of fire roasted tomatoes
1 ½ cup (about 1) roasted red pepper
½ onion, roughly chopped
2 cloves garlic
1 tablespoons maple syrup
Salt and pepper to taste

Combine all ingredients in blender. Blend until smooth.

Miss O's Seasoned Salt:
Ingredients:
4 tablespoon sea salt
2 tablespoon onion powder
2 tablespoon garlic powder
2 tablespoon paprika
2 tablespoon celery salt
2 tablespoon coconut sugar
2 tablespoon black pepper
1 ½ teaspoon cayenne
2 teaspoon turmeric

Directions:
Combine all ingredients. Store in an airtight container.

EASY SALAD DRESSING MATRIX

Directions:
Choose 1 Oil, 1 vinegar, 1 teaspoon salt, and add herbs and spices to your heart's content!

Add to a blender to combine. Tastes best when allowed to rest refrigerated for an hour or more. Store in an airtight container.

3/4 cup oil	1/4 cup vinegar	Herb/Spice 1 teaspoon (adjust to taste)	Additions 1 Tablespoon (adjust to taste)
Olive Oil	Apple Cider (mild - universal)	Basil	Raw Honey
Avocado Oil	Balsamic (sweet - universal)	Parsley	Dijon Mustard
Macadamia Nut Oil	Red Wine (hearty - beef/pork)	Rosemary	Minced Scallions
Walnut Oil	White Wine (light - poultry/fish)	Thyme	Minced Red Onion
Hazelnut Oil	Champagne (light - poultry/fish)	Oregano	Bacon
	Rice Wine (very mild - low acid)	Dill	Lemon Juice
		White Pepper	1 hard boiled egg (creamier vinaigrette)
		Garlic Powder	
		Onion Powder	
		Red Pepper Flakes	
		Dried Chives	
		Dry Mustard	

Easy Italian dressing: Olive Oil, Apple Cider Vinegar, Basil, Parsley, Rosemary, Oregano, Garlic Powder, Red Pepper Flakes.

The Tao of Paleo

The Tao of Paleo

ABOUT JASON AND JOE

Jason Goldberg is a writer, blogger, mud racer, martial artist, and a heavy metal transport specialist. He mentors newcomers to the paleo lifestyle through his Paleo Padawan program. His first novel, *Pilot Error,* will be published in early 2015. He lives on the East Coast with his son, Joseph, and a sun conure named Woodstock.

Joe Salama is the publisher, co-editor, and contributing author of The Paleo Miracle: 50 Real Stories of Health Transformation, the producer of the Ancestral Food Summit, contributing writer for Paleo Movement Online Magazine, and one of the Administrators of the International Paleo Movement Group on Facebook. Joe earned two Bachelor of Arts degrees from University of California at Berkeley, one in Rhetoric, one in Economics, a law degree from Boston University, and a mediation certification from U.C. Berkeley. He is a father, a trial attorney, mediator, paleo missionary man, author, skydiver, charity fundraiser, choy li fut kung fu practitioner, and sits on the board of directors of several non-profits including The Paleo Foundation.

The Tao of Paleo